THE MIND DIET COOKBOOK

150+ Nutrient-rich recipes to boost brain health, enhance cognitive function and fuel your mind for a vibrant life

TERESA MILLER

COPYRIGHT ©
All rights reserved.

No part of this book may be reproduced in any form or by any electronic or mechanical means, including information storage and retrieval systems, without permission in writing from the publisher, except by a reviewer who may quote brief passages in a review.

The information contained in this book is based on the author's research and experience. While the author has made every effort to provide accurate and up-to-date information, errors and omissions may occur. The author and publisher assume no responsibility for any errors or omissions or for any actions taken based on the information contained in this book.

The information contained in this book is provided "as is," without warranty of any kind, express or implied, including but not limited to the warranties of merchantability, fitness for a particular purpose, or non-infringement. In no event shall the author or publisher be liable for any claim, damages, or other liability, whether in an action of contract, tort, or otherwise, arising from, out of, or in connection with the book or the use or other dealings in the book.

TABLE OF CONTENTS

CHAPTER THREE--152

INTRODUCTION

In the hustle and bustle of modern life, our minds are the silent warriors navigating through an incessant influx of information, tasks, and responsibilities. The concept of wellness has evolved beyond the mere sustenance of our bodies; it encompasses nurturing our mental faculties to ensure clarity, focus, and resilience. Enter the Mind Diet – an intriguing approach not just for bodily nourishment but also for the profound care and fortification of our most vital organ: the brain.

The Mind Diet stands as a nutritional compass, guiding individuals toward food choices that not only satiate hunger but also foster cognitive prowess and shield against cognitive decline. Originating from a fusion of the Mediterranean and DASH (Dietary Approaches to Stop Hypertension) diets, this approach champions an assortment of wholesome, brain-boosting foods that form the cornerstone of a dietary strategy primed for neurological health.

At its core, the Mind Diet espouses the power of specific nutrients, antioxidants, and healthy fats found abundantly in certain food groups. These nutritional elements have been scientifically linked to reducing the risk of cognitive impairment, Alzheimer's disease, and other forms of cognitive decline. Embracing this philosophy transcends the mere act of eating; it embodies a proactive stance towards safeguarding our cognitive well-being through mindful consumption.

The Mind Diet's design is strategic, integrating foods rich in brain-loving nutrients such as omega-3 fatty acids, antioxidants, and vitamins crucial for neural resilience. Its emphasis on leafy greens, whole grains, nuts, berries, fish, and olive oil contributes to a culinary palette celebrated for its multifaceted benefits. Studies have underscored the correlation between adherence to the Mind Diet and improved cognitive function, making it a beacon of hope in the quest for long-term brain health.

By cultivating a diet replete with these nourishing elements, individuals embark on a journey toward not just the gratification of taste buds but also the preservation of cognitive sharpness and vitality. The Mind Diet is not a fleeting trend but a sustainable lifestyle choice that champions the longevity and vitality of the mind. The Mind Diet doesn't merely promise culinary satisfaction; it offers a roadmap to potentially enhancing memory, sharpening focus, and nurturing a healthier, more vibrant brain as we navigate the chapters of life.

In this guide, we unravel the intricate tapestry of the Mind Diet, offering a treasure trove of delectable recipes, insightful nutritional information, and practical tips to empower you on your path to a nourished mind and a thriving life. Prepare to embark on a gastronomic adventure that celebrates the union of tantalizing flavors and the profound nourishment of your most invaluable asset - your brain.

Welcome to the Mind Diet Cookbook - where culinary delight meets cognitive fortification.

CHAPTER ONE

THE MIND DIET'S BACKGROUND

The Mind Diet, short for "Mediterranean-DASH Intervention for Neurodegenerative Delay," was developed as a dietary approach specifically aimed at promoting brain health and reducing the risk of cognitive decline, particularly conditions like Alzheimer's disease.

Origins:

The Mind Diet draws its foundations from two well-established dietary patterns:

• Mediterranean Diet:

Originating from the Mediterranean region, this diet emphasizes whole, plant-based foods such as fruits, vegetables, whole grains, nuts, seeds, and olive oil. It also includes moderate consumption of fish, poultry, and dairy while limiting red meat and processed foods.

• DASH Diet (Dietary Approaches to Stop Hypertension):

Initially designed to help manage high blood pressure, the DASH Diet emphasizes fruits, vegetables, lean proteins, whole grains, and low-fat dairy while reducing sodium intake.

Development:

Researchers noticed that both the Mediterranean and DASH diets individually showed promise in promoting heart health and reducing the risk of chronic diseases. Building on these findings, they sought to create a dietary plan that specifically targeted brain health and cognitive function.

Purpose and Goals:

The primary aim of the Mind Diet is to provide a nutritional strategy that combines elements from these two diets to optimize brain health. It focuses on incorporating foods that are rich in nutrients believed to support cognitive function, such as:

• Antioxidants: Found in fruits, vegetables, and certain spices, antioxidants help combat oxidative stress, which may contribute to brain aging.

• Omega-3 Fatty Acids: Abundant in fatty fish like salmon, as well as in nuts and seeds, these healthy fats are linked to better brain health and cognitive function.

• Vitamins and Minerals: Nutrients like vitamin E, vitamin B12, and folate are thought to be crucial for brain health and are found in various foods like leafy greens, nuts, and legumes.

Scientific Support:

Numerous studies have investigated the Mind Diet's potential benefits for brain health. Some research suggests that adhering to the Mind Diet may lower the risk of developing Alzheimer's disease and slow cognitive decline in older adults. However, more extensive and long-term studies are ongoing to further validate these findings.

Implementation:

The Mind Diet emphasizes a balanced and diverse selection of whole, nutrient-rich foods while reducing the intake of processed foods, red meat, and sweets. Its approach aims to provide a sustainable and enjoyable dietary pattern that supports not only brain health but overall well-being.

This dietary approach continues to garner attention in the field of nutrition and cognitive health as researchers delve deeper into understanding the relationship between diet and brain function, offering hope for a proactive approach to maintaining cognitive vitality throughout life.

THE MIND DIET'S PHILOSOPHY

The philosophy of the Mind Diet revolves around the belief that the foods we consume can significantly impact our brain health and cognitive function over time. Its core principles are rooted in the idea that a well-balanced and nutrient-rich diet can potentially reduce the risk of cognitive decline, protect against neurodegenerative diseases, and promote long-term brain health.

Key Tenets of the Mind Diet Philosophy:

• Nutrient-Dense Foods: The Mind Diet places a strong emphasis on consuming nutrient-dense foods, particularly those that are rich in specific nutrients known to support brain health. This includes antioxidants, omega-3 fatty acids, vitamins, and minerals that may offer protection against cognitive decline and support optimal brain function.

• Whole, Plant-Based Foods: The foundation of the Mind Diet is built upon a variety of whole, plant-based foods such as fruits, vegetables, whole grains, nuts, seeds, and legumes. These foods are packed with essential nutrients and antioxidants believed to have positive effects on brain health.

• Moderation and Balance: While promoting the consumption of beneficial foods, the Mind Diet also encourages moderation in the intake of certain food groups. It suggests moderate consumption of lean proteins, particularly fish and poultry, and limited intake of red meat, processed foods, and sweets.

• Long-Term Health Benefits: The philosophy of the Mind Diet extends beyond immediate health benefits, aiming to establish a dietary pattern that supports long-term brain health and reduces the risk of cognitive decline as individuals age.

• Lifestyle Approach: It advocates for a holistic approach to health that combines diet with other lifestyle factors such as regular physical activity, mental stimulation, social engagement, and adequate sleep – all contributing to overall brain health and cognitive resilience.

• Adaptability and Enjoyment: The Mind Diet is designed to be adaptable and flexible, allowing individuals to personalize their meals while enjoying a diverse range of flavorful and nutritious foods. This adaptability aims to make it easier for individuals to adopt and sustain this dietary approach as part of their lifestyle.

Implementation and Practicality:

The Mind Diet's philosophy doesn't promote deprivation or extreme dietary changes. Instead, it encourages a balanced and enjoyable approach to eating, emphasizing the inclusion of beneficial foods while gradually reducing less healthy choices. By focusing on nutrient-rich foods and minimizing processed and unhealthy options, it aims to create a sustainable and practical dietary pattern that supports cognitive health throughout life.

In essence, the Mind Diet philosophy promotes the idea that what we eat matters not only for our physical health but also for the vitality and resilience of our brains, offering a proactive way to nourish and protect our cognitive well-being as we age.

The Mind Diet is specifically designed to support brain health through its emphasis on certain nutrient-rich foods and the avoidance of potentially harmful dietary elements. Here's how the Mind Diet supports brain health:

• Protects Against Oxidative Stress: Antioxidants found in fruits, vegetables, and herbs combat oxidative stress, reducing cellular damage in the brain. This protection may help prevent age-related cognitive decline and neurodegenerative diseases.

• Enhances Brain Function: Foods high in omega-3 fatty acids like fatty fish (salmon, mackerel) and nuts are believed to support brain health. They contribute to improved cognitive function, potentially reducing the risk of dementia and improving memory.

• Reduces Inflammation: The Mind Diet's focus on whole grains, nuts, and fruits with anti-inflammatory properties helps reduce inflammation in the body, which can be linked to brain health. Chronic inflammation may contribute to neurodegenerative diseases.

• Promotes Healthy Circulation: By incorporating heart-healthy foods like olive oil, the Mind Diet supports good blood flow, ensuring the brain receives a steady supply of oxygen and nutrients vital for optimal function.

• Vitamins and Minerals: Foods like leafy greens, berries, nuts, and beans are rich in vitamins (e.g., vitamin E, B vitamins) and minerals (e.g., folate) that are crucial for brain health and cognitive function.

• Limits Unhealthy Fats and Sugars: Reducing the intake of saturated fats, trans fats, and excessive sugars, commonly found in processed and fried foods, may help mitigate the risk of cognitive decline and support overall brain health.

• Focus on Lifestyle Factors: The Mind Diet doesn't solely emphasize food; it encourages a holistic approach to health. Regular exercise, mental stimulation, social engagement, and quality sleep complement dietary efforts and further support brain health.

• Scientific Studies: Research has shown that adherence to the Mind Diet is associated with slower cognitive decline, improved cognitive function, and a reduced risk of developing Alzheimer's disease or other forms of dementia.

• Promotes Long-Term Health: The Mind Diet advocates for a sustainable dietary pattern that can be adopted and maintained over the long term, providing ongoing support for brain health throughout one's life.

In summary, the Mind Diet's emphasis on specific nutrient-rich foods, combined with its avoidance of potentially detrimental dietary elements, creates a dietary pattern that supports brain health, potentially reducing the risk of cognitive decline and promoting overall cognitive well-being.

Several nutrients play vital roles in supporting brain health and cognitive function. Here are some key nutrients and their contributions to brain health:

1. Omega-3 Fatty Acids:

• Function: Essential for building and maintaining brain cell membranes, aiding in communication between brain cells, and reducing inflammation.

• Sources: Fatty fish (salmon, mackerel, sardines), flaxseeds, chia seeds, walnuts.

2. Antioxidants:

• Function: Protect brain cells from oxidative stress and damage caused by free radicals, potentially reducing the risk of cognitive decline.

• Sources: Colorful fruits and vegetables (berries, spinach, kale, broccoli), herbs (turmeric, cinnamon), nuts, and seeds.

3. Vitamin E:

• Function: Acts as an antioxidant, protecting cell membranes from oxidative damage, potentially reducing the risk of Alzheimer's disease.

• Sources: Nuts (almonds, sunflower seeds), seeds, spinach, avocado, vegetable oils.

4. Vitamin C:

• Function: Enhances the immune system, aids in the production of neurotransmitters, and supports brain health through its antioxidant properties.

• Sources: Citrus fruits (oranges, lemons), strawberries, bell peppers, broccoli.

5. B Vitamins (B6, B9 - Folate, B12):

• Function: Essential for neurotransmitter synthesis, DNA repair, and the production of red blood cells crucial for oxygen transport to the brain.

• Sources: Leafy greens, legumes, fortified cereals, eggs, dairy, poultry, fish.

6. Vitamin D:

• Function: Supports brain development, cognitive function, and may protect against cognitive decline.

• Sources: Sunlight exposure, fatty fish (salmon, tuna), fortified dairy products, fortified cereals.

7. Magnesium:

• Function: Involved in neurotransmitter function, supports brain plasticity, and helps regulate nerve and muscle function.

• Sources: Whole grains, nuts, seeds, leafy greens, legumes.

8. Zinc:

• Function: Supports neurotransmitter function, aids in learning and memory, and contributes to overall brain health.

• Sources: Shellfish, red meat, poultry, beans, nuts, whole grains.

9. Iron:

• Function: Essential for oxygen transport to the brain, energy production, and cognitive function.

• Sources: Red meat, poultry, fish, lentils, beans, fortified cereals.

10. Phospholipids and Choline:

• Function: Crucial for brain cell membrane structure and function, neurotransmitter synthesis, and cognitive development.

• Sources: Eggs, liver, soybeans, peanuts, certain fish (salmon).

These nutrients work synergistically to support various aspects of brain health, including cognitive function, memory, mood regulation, and overall neurological well-being. A balanced diet rich in a variety of nutrient-dense foods is essential for ensuring an adequate intake of these nutrients to support optimal brain health throughout life.

LISTS OF RECOMMENDED FOODS AND THOSE TO LIMIT OR AVOID ON THE MIND DIET

The Mind Diet emphasizes the consumption of nutrient-rich foods that support brain health while recommending limitations on certain less beneficial foods. Here are comprehensive lists of recommended foods and those to limit or avoid on the Mind Diet:

Recommended Foods on the Mind Diet:

Fruits:

• Berries (blueberries, strawberries, raspberries)

• Citrus fruits (oranges, lemons, grapefruits)

• Apples

• Avocados

• Bananas

• Grapes

Vegetables:

• Leafy greens (spinach, kale, Swiss chard)

• Broccoli

• Brussels sprouts

- Cauliflower

- Bell peppers (red, yellow, green)

- Carrots

Whole Grains:

- Oats

- Brown rice

- Quinoa

- Whole grain bread and pasta

- Barley

- Bulgur

Nuts and Seeds:

- Almonds

- Walnuts

- Flaxseeds

- Chia seeds

- Sunflower seeds

- Pumpkin seeds

Legumes:

• Beans (black beans, kidney beans, chickpeas)

• Lentils

• Peas

Fish and Seafood:

• Fatty fish (salmon, mackerel, sardines, trout)

• Shellfish (shrimp, oysters)

Poultry:

• Chicken

• Turkey

Dairy and Alternatives:

• Low-fat dairy products (yogurt, milk, cheese)

• Plant-based milk alternatives (almond milk, oat milk, soy milk)

Healthy Fats:

• Olive oil

• Avocado oil

• Nuts and seeds

Herbs and Spices:

• Turmeric

• Cinnamon

• Ginger

• Rosemary

• Oregano

• Basil

Foods to Limit or Avoid on the Mind Diet:

Red Meat:

• Beef

• Lamb

• Pork

Processed and Fried Foods:

• Fast food

• Processed meats (sausages, bacon)

• Fried foods (french fries, fried chicken)

Full-Fat Dairy and Butter:

• High-fat cheeses

• Full-fat butter

Sweets and Sugary Beverages:

• Candies

• Pastries

• Soda

• Sweetened beverages

Trans Fats and Partially Hydrogenated Oils:

• Margarine

• Processed snacks with trans fats

Excessive Salt:

• High-sodium processed foods

• Salty snacks

The Mind Diet encourages the regular consumption of the recommended foods rich in antioxidants, omega-3 fatty acids, and essential nutrients while minimizing or avoiding foods high in saturated fats, added sugars, and processed ingredients that may have adverse effects on brain health over time.

METHODS THAT MAINTAIN THE NUTRITIONAL INTEGRITY OF THE INGREDIENTS AND MAXIMIZE THEIR BENEFITS

Maintaining the nutritional integrity of ingredients and maximizing their benefits involves various cooking and preparation methods that preserve nutrients while enhancing their bioavailability. Here are methods to consider:

Cooking Techniques:

Steaming:

• Retains water-soluble vitamins like vitamin C and B vitamins.

• Preserves color, texture, and nutrients in vegetables.

Stir-Frying:

• Quick cooking at high heat helps retain nutrients.

• Use minimal oil and cook vegetables briefly to maintain crunchiness.

Sautéing:

• Use low to medium heat and minimal oil to preserve nutrients.

• Quick cooking helps retain flavor and nutrients in vegetables.

Grilling or Broiling:

• Retains nutrients and imparts a smoky flavor to food.

• Use lean cuts of meat, fish, or vegetables to minimize fat drippings.

Baking or Roasting:

• Preserves nutrients by cooking food in its juices.

• Cook vegetables and meats at moderate temperatures to retain nutrients.

Food Preparation Tips:

• Preserve Vegetable Peels: Many nutrients are concentrated in the peels of fruits and vegetables. Wash thoroughly and consider leaving the peels on when appropriate.

• Minimal Processing: Avoid excessive chopping, cutting, or peeling, which can lead to nutrient loss. Opt for whole fruits and vegetables as much as possible.

• Proper Storage: Store fruits and vegetables properly to retain their nutrients. Refrigerate or store in a cool, dark place to prevent nutrient degradation.

• Use Healthy Cooking Oils: Use oils rich in unsaturated fats like olive oil or avocado oil for cooking. These oils preserve nutrients and provide healthy fats.

Maximizing Nutrient Absorption:

• Pairing Foods: Combine certain foods to enhance nutrient absorption. For example, pairing foods rich in vitamin C (like citrus fruits) with iron-rich foods (like spinach) can improve iron absorption.

• Include Healthy Fats: Adding healthy fats to meals can aid in the absorption of fat-soluble vitamins (A, D, E, K) found in vegetables. For instance, adding olive oil to salads can enhance the absorption of fat-soluble nutrients.

• Consider Raw Options: Some nutrients are better preserved in their raw form. Include a variety of raw fruits, vegetables, and nuts in your diet to benefit from their natural nutrients.

Avoid Overcooking:

• Limit Boiling: Boiling vegetables can lead to nutrient loss due to leaching into the water. If using water, consider using it in soups or stews to retain the nutrients.

• Cook Just Enough: Avoid prolonged cooking times, as they can cause nutrient degradation. Cook until foods are tender but not overly soft.

Balancing these methods while preparing meals can help maintain the nutritional integrity of ingredients and optimize the health benefits derived from the foods consumed.

COOKING TIPS WHEN FOLLOWING THE MIND DIET

When following the Mind Diet, certain cooking tips can help maximize the nutritional benefits of the foods you consume. Here are cooking tips tailored to support the principles of the Mind Diet:

Emphasize Plant-Based Ingredients:

Tip 1: Focus on Fresh Produce

• Use a variety of colorful fruits and vegetables in your meals. Opt for fresh, whole produce to maximize nutrient intake.

Tip 2: Lightly Cook or Enjoy Raw

• Consider lightly steaming or sautéing vegetables to retain their nutrients. Eating some vegetables raw can also preserve their natural goodness.

Tip 3: Experiment with Herbs and Spices

• Use herbs and spices generously to add flavor without relying on excessive salt or unhealthy seasonings.

Include Brain-Boosting Omega-3s:

Tip 1: Choose Fatty Fish Wisely

• Opt for cooking methods that preserve the omega-3 fatty acids in fish, such as baking, grilling, or steaming. Avoid excessive frying to retain the nutrients.

Tip 2: Incorporate Plant-Based Sources

• Include flaxseeds, chia seeds, and walnuts in your diet by adding them to salads, smoothies, or as toppings for yogurt or oatmeal.

Whole Grains and Legumes:

Tip 1: Opt for Whole Grain Varieties

• Choose whole grain options like brown rice, quinoa, and whole grain pasta. These can be cooked by methods such as boiling or steaming to retain nutrients.

Tip 2: Experiment with Legumes

• Cook beans and lentils using methods like boiling or pressure cooking, and incorporate them into soups, stews, or salads.

Lean Proteins:

Tip 1: Choose Lean Cuts of Meat

• Trim visible fat from meat before cooking and use healthier cooking methods like grilling, baking, or broiling.

Tip 2: Try Poultry and Plant-Based Proteins

• Experiment with lean poultry cuts, such as chicken or turkey, and explore plant-based protein sources like tofu, tempeh, or legumes.

Healthy Cooking Practices:

Tip 1: Minimize Oil Usage

• Use heart-healthy oils like olive oil or avocado oil sparingly to preserve nutrients and enhance flavors.

Tip 2: Avoid Overcooking

• Cook foods until just tender to avoid nutrient loss. Overcooking vegetables or proteins can reduce their nutritional content.

Tip 3: Be Mindful of Portion Sizes

• Practice portion control to ensure a balanced intake of nutrients without overindulging in any particular food group.

By incorporating these cooking tips into your meal preparation, you can maintain the nutritional quality of your foods while following the Mind Diet's principles, promoting brain health and overall well-being.

CHAPTER TWO

BREAKFAST RECIPES

Berry and Spinach Smoothie Bowl

Ingredients:

• 1 cup fresh spinach leaves

• 1 ripe banana

• 1/2 cup mixed berries (strawberries, blueberries, raspberries)

• 1/2 cup plain Greek yogurt

• 1 tablespoon chia seeds

• 1/4 cup almond milk (or any preferred milk)

• Toppings: sliced almonds, shredded coconut, additional berries

Instructions:

1. Wash the spinach leaves and berries thoroughly. Slice the banana.

2. In a blender, combine the spinach, banana, mixed berries, Greek yogurt, chia seeds, and almond milk.

3. Blend until smooth and creamy.

4. Pour the smoothie into a bowl. Top with sliced almonds, shredded coconut, and additional berries for added texture and flavor.

Avocado and Smoked Salmon Toast

Ingredients:

• 2 slices whole grain bread

• 1 ripe avocado

• 100g smoked salmon

• 1 tablespoon lemon juice

• Fresh dill or parsley for garnish

• Salt and pepper to taste

Instructions:

1. Toast the whole grain bread slices to your desired level of crispness.

2. Mash the ripe avocado in a bowl. Mix in lemon juice, salt, and pepper.

3. Spread the mashed avocado evenly onto the toasted bread slices. Layer smoked salmon on top of the avocado.

4. Garnish with fresh dill or parsley.

Greek Yogurt Parfait with Mixed Berries and Granola

Ingredients:

- 1 cup plain Greek yogurt

- 1/2 cup mixed berries (blueberries, strawberries)

- 1/4 cup granola (low-sugar, whole grain)

Instructions:

1. In a glass or bowl, start by adding a layer of Greek yogurt.

2. Top the yogurt layer with mixed berries. Sprinkle a layer of granola over the berries.

3. Repeat the layering process with the remaining yogurt, berries, and granola.

Spinach and Feta Egg Muffins

Ingredients:

- 6 large eggs

- 1 cup fresh spinach (chopped)

• 1/4 cup crumbled feta cheese

• Salt and pepper to taste

• Cooking spray or olive oil for greasing muffin tin

Instructions:

1. Preheat the oven to 350°F (175°C). Grease a muffin tin with cooking spray or olive oil.

2. In a mixing bowl, whisk together eggs, chopped spinach, crumbled feta cheese, salt, and pepper.

3. Pour the egg mixture evenly into the prepared muffin cups, filling each about 3/4 full.

4. Bake in the preheated oven for 20-25 minutes or until the egg muffins are set and lightly golden.

Overnight Oats with Berries and Almonds

Ingredients:

• 1/2 cup rolled oats

• 1/2 cup almond milk (or any preferred milk)

• 1 tablespoon chia seeds

• 1/4 cup mixed berries (blueberries, raspberries)

• 1 tablespoon sliced almonds

• 1 teaspoon honey or maple syrup (optional for sweetness)

Instructions:

1. In a jar or container, mix rolled oats, almond milk, chia seeds, mixed berries, sliced almonds, and honey or maple syrup if desired.

2. Cover the jar or container and refrigerate the mixture overnight or for at least 4 hours.

3. Stir the mixture before serving and enjoy cold or at room temperature in the morning.

Veggie Omelette with Spinach and Tomatoes

Ingredients:

• 3 large eggs

• 1 cup fresh spinach (chopped)

• 1/2 cup cherry tomatoes (halved)

• 1/4 cup diced bell peppers

• 2 tablespoons diced onion

• 1 tablespoon olive oil

- Salt and pepper to taste

- Optional: Feta cheese or herbs for garnish

Instructions:

1. Heat olive oil in a non-stick skillet over medium heat.

2. Sauté diced onions, bell peppers, and cherry tomatoes until slightly softened.

3. In a bowl, whisk the eggs and season with salt and pepper. Add chopped spinach to the egg mixture and combine.

4. Pour the egg and spinach mixture into the skillet over the sautéed vegetables. Allow the eggs to cook until the edges set, then gently fold the omelette in half.

5. Cook for another minute or until the eggs are fully cooked through.

6. Slide the omelette onto a plate and garnish with optional feta cheese or herbs.

Quinoa Breakfast Bowl with Berries and Almonds

Ingredients:

- 1/2 cup cooked quinoa

- 1/4 cup almond milk (or any preferred milk)

- 1 tablespoon honey or maple syrup

- 1/4 cup mixed berries (strawberries, blueberries)

- 1 tablespoon sliced almonds

- Cinnamon for sprinkling (optional)

Instructions:

1. In a bowl, combine cooked quinoa, almond milk, honey or maple syrup, and mix well.

2. Top the quinoa mixture with mixed berries and sliced almonds. Sprinkle with cinnamon if desired.

3. Gently mix the ingredients together and enjoy the quinoa breakfast bowl.

Mediterranean Breakfast Toast with Hummus and Tomatoes

Ingredients:

- 2 slices whole grain bread (toasted)

- 1/4 cup hummus

- 1/2 cup cherry tomatoes (halved)

- Fresh basil leaves for garnish

• Olive oil for drizzling

• Salt and pepper to taste

Instructions:

1. Toast the whole grain bread slices until golden brown.

2. Spread hummus evenly onto the toasted bread slices. Arrange halved cherry tomatoes on top of the hummus.

3. Garnish with fresh basil leaves. Drizzle a bit of olive oil over the tomatoes.

4. Sprinkle with salt and pepper to taste.

Chia Seed Pudding with Mixed Fruit

Ingredients:

• 1/4 cup chia seeds

• 1 cup almond milk (or any preferred milk)

• 1 tablespoon honey or maple syrup

• 1/2 cup mixed fruit (sliced strawberries, kiwi, mango)

• Sliced almonds or shredded coconut for topping

Instructions:

1. In a bowl, combine chia seeds, almond milk, and honey or maple syrup.

2. Stir well to combine and let it sit for 5 minutes. Stir again to prevent clumping.

3. Cover the bowl and refrigerate the chia seed mixture overnight or for at least 4 hours to allow it to thicken.

4. Stir the chia seed pudding mixture and divide it into serving bowls.

5. Top with mixed fruit slices, sliced almonds, or shredded coconut.

Spinach and Mushroom Breakfast Frittata

Ingredients:

• 6 large eggs

• 1 cup fresh spinach leaves

• 1/2 cup sliced mushrooms

• 1/4 cup diced onion

• 1/4 cup shredded mozzarella cheese

- 1 tablespoon olive oil

- Salt and pepper to taste

Instructions:

1. Preheat the oven to 350°F (175°C).

2. In an oven-safe skillet, heat olive oil over medium heat.

3. Sauté diced onions until translucent, then add sliced mushrooms and spinach. Cook until spinach wilts.

4. In a bowl, whisk eggs and season with salt and pepper. Pour the whisked eggs over the sautéed vegetables in the skillet.

5. Sprinkle shredded mozzarella cheese evenly over the egg mixture.

6. Transfer the skillet to the preheated oven and bake for 15-20 minutes or until the frittata is set and lightly golden on top.

7. Slice the frittata into wedges and serve hot.

Almond Butter and Banana Overnight Oats

Ingredients:

- 1/2 cup rolled oats

- 1 cup almond milk (or any preferred milk)

- 2 tablespoons almond butter

- 1 ripe banana (sliced)

- 1 tablespoon honey or maple syrup (optional)

- Sliced almonds for topping

Instructions:

1. In a jar or container, mix rolled oats, almond milk, almond butter, and honey or maple syrup if desired.

2. Add sliced banana into the mixture and stir well.

3. Cover the jar or container and refrigerate the mixture overnight or for at least 4 hours.

4. Stir the mixture before serving and sprinkle sliced almonds on top.

Mediterranean Avocado Toast with Poached Egg

Ingredients:

- 2 slices whole grain bread (toasted)

- 1 ripe avocado

- 2 eggs

- Cherry tomatoes (sliced)

- Fresh basil leaves for garnish

- Olive oil for drizzling

- Salt and pepper to taste

Instructions:

1. Toast the whole grain bread slices until golden brown. Mash the ripe avocado in a bowl and season with salt and pepper.

2. Fill a pot with water and bring it to a gentle simmer.

3. Crack eggs into the simmering water and poach for about 3-4 minutes until the whites are set.

4. Spread the mashed avocado onto the toasted bread slices. Top each toast with a poached egg.

5. Add sliced cherry tomatoes and garnish with fresh basil leaves.

6. Drizzle olive oil and sprinkle with salt and pepper.

Blueberry and Walnut Breakfast Quinoa

Ingredients:

• 1/2 cup cooked quinoa

• 1/4 cup almond milk (or any preferred milk)

• 1/2 cup fresh blueberries

• 2 tablespoons chopped walnuts

• 1 tablespoon honey or maple syrup

• Cinnamon for sprinkling (optional)

Instructions:

1. In a bowl, combine cooked quinoa, almond milk, honey or maple syrup, and mix well.

2. Top the quinoa mixture with fresh blueberries and chopped walnuts. Sprinkle with cinnamon if desired.

3. Gently mix the ingredients together and enjoy the nutritious quinoa bowl.

Spinach and Mushroom Breakfast Burrito

Ingredients:

- 2 large whole grain tortillas

- 4 eggs (scrambled)

- 1 cup fresh spinach leaves

- 1/2 cup sliced mushrooms

- 1/4 cup shredded cheddar cheese

- 2 tablespoons salsa

- Cooking spray or olive oil for cooking

Instructions:

1. In a skillet, heat cooking spray or olive oil over medium heat.

2. Sauté sliced mushrooms until they start to brown, then add fresh spinach and cook until wilted.

3. Scramble eggs in a separate pan until cooked. Warm tortillas briefly in the microwave or on a skillet.

4. Layer scrambled eggs, sautéed vegetables, shredded cheddar cheese, and salsa onto each tortilla.

5. Roll the tortillas into burritos, tucking in the sides. Serve immediately or wrap in foil for an on-the-go breakfast.

Greek Yogurt and Berry Breakfast Popsicles

Ingredients:

• 1 cup Greek yogurt

• 1/2 cup mixed berries (blueberries, strawberries)

• 1 tablespoon honey or maple syrup

• Popsicle molds and sticks

Instructions:

1. In a bowl, mix Greek yogurt with honey or maple syrup until well combined.

2. Add mixed berries into the yogurt mixture and stir gently.

3. Spoon the yogurt and berry mixture into popsicle molds. Insert popsicle sticks into each mold.

4. Place the popsicle molds in the freezer and let them freeze for at least 4-6 hours or until solid.

5. Remove the popsicles from the molds and enjoy these refreshing breakfast treats.

Sweet Potato and Spinach Breakfast Hash

Ingredients:

• 2 medium sweet potatoes (peeled and diced)

• 1 cup fresh spinach (chopped)

• 1/2 cup diced bell peppers

• 1/4 cup diced onion

• 2 cloves garlic (minced)

• 2 eggs

• 2 tablespoons olive oil

• Salt, pepper, and paprika to taste

Instructions:

1. Heat olive oil in a skillet over medium heat.

2. Add diced sweet potatoes and cook until they begin to soften. Add diced bell peppers, onions, and minced garlic. Sauté until vegetables are tender.

3. Season with salt, pepper, and paprika to taste.

4. Stir in chopped spinach and cook until wilted.

5. Create two wells in the hash and crack an egg into each well. Cover the skillet and cook until the eggs are cooked to your liking.

6. Divide the hash and eggs onto plates and enjoy.

Whole Grain Pancakes with Berries

Ingredients:

• 1 cup whole wheat flour

• 1 tablespoon baking powder

• 1 tablespoon honey or maple syrup

• 1 cup almond milk (or any preferred milk)

• 1 egg

• Mixed berries for topping

• Greek yogurt for serving (optional)

Instructions:

1. In a mixing bowl, whisk together whole wheat flour and baking powder.

2. Add honey or maple syrup, almond milk, and egg. Mix until smooth.

3. Heat a non-stick skillet over medium heat and lightly grease with cooking spray or oil.

4. Pour 1/4 cup of batter onto the skillet for each pancake. Cook until bubbles form on the surface, then flip and cook until golden brown.

5. Stack the pancakes and top with mixed berries. Optionally, serve with a dollop of Greek yogurt.

Tofu Scramble with Vegetables

Ingredients:

- 1 block firm tofu (pressed and crumbled)

- 1 cup diced bell peppers

- 1/2 cup diced tomatoes

- 1/4 cup diced onion

- 2 cloves garlic (minced)

- 1 tablespoon nutritional yeast (optional)

- 2 tablespoons olive oil

- Salt, pepper, and turmeric to taste

Instructions:

1. Heat olive oil in a skillet over medium heat.

2. Sauté diced onions and minced garlic until fragrant. Add diced bell peppers and tomatoes, cook until softened.

3. Add crumbled tofu to the skillet and stir well.

4. Season with salt, pepper, turmeric, and nutritional yeast (if using). Mix until tofu is evenly coated and heated through.

5. Transfer the tofu scramble to plates and enjoy.

Apple Cinnamon Overnight Chia Pudding

Ingredients:

• 1/4 cup chia seeds

• 1 cup almond milk (or any preferred milk)

• 1 tablespoon honey or maple syrup

• 1 apple (peeled, cored, and diced)

• 1/2 teaspoon ground cinnamon

• Sliced almonds for topping

Instructions:

1. In a bowl or jar, combine chia seeds, almond milk, honey or maple syrup, diced apple, and cinnamon. Stir well.

2. Cover and refrigerate the mixture overnight or for at least 4 hours to thicken.

3. Stir the chia pudding and portion into bowls. Top with sliced almonds before serving.

Spinach and Mushroom Egg Muffin Cups

Ingredients:

• 6 eggs

• 1 cup fresh spinach (chopped)

• 1/2 cup sliced mushrooms

• 1/4 cup diced onion

• 1/4 cup shredded mozzarella cheese

• Cooking spray or olive oil for greasing muffin tin

• Salt, pepper, and herbs of choice (optional)

Instructions:

1. Preheat the oven to 350°F (175°C).

2. In a bowl, whisk eggs and season with salt, pepper, and herbs if using.

3. Stir in chopped spinach, sliced mushrooms, diced onion, and shredded mozzarella cheese.

4. Grease a muffin tin with cooking spray or olive oil. Pour the egg mixture evenly into the prepared muffin cups.

5. Bake in the preheated oven for 20-25 minutes or until the egg muffin cups are set.

6. Allow the egg muffin cups to cool slightly before removing them from the tin. Serve warm.

Berry Spinach Breakfast Salad

Ingredients:

• 2 cups fresh spinach leaves

• 1/2 cup mixed berries (strawberries, blueberries, raspberries)

• 1/4 cup sliced almonds

• 2 tablespoons crumbled feta cheese

• Balsamic vinaigrette dressing

Instructions:

1. Wash and dry the spinach leaves thoroughly.

2. Slice the strawberries and prepare other berries as desired.

3. In a bowl, combine fresh spinach, mixed berries, sliced almonds, and crumbled feta cheese.

4. Drizzle balsamic vinaigrette dressing over the salad just before serving.

Egg and Vegetable Breakfast Wrap

Ingredients:

• 2 large eggs

• 2 whole grain wraps or tortillas

• 1/2 cup diced bell peppers (mixed colors)

• 1/4 cup diced onion

• 1/2 cup fresh spinach leaves

• 1/4 cup shredded mozzarella cheese

• Cooking spray or olive oil

- Salt, pepper, and herbs of choice (optional)

Instructions:

1. In a skillet, heat cooking spray or olive oil over medium heat.

2. Sauté diced bell peppers and onions until softened, then add spinach and cook until wilted.

3. Whisk eggs in a bowl, season with salt, pepper, and herbs if desired, and scramble in the skillet with the vegetables.

4. Warm the wraps or tortillas. Spread the scrambled egg and vegetable mixture onto each wrap.

5. Sprinkle shredded mozzarella cheese on top.

6. Roll up the wraps, folding in the sides, and serve immediately.

Blueberry Almond Butter Toast

Ingredients:

- 2 slices whole grain bread (toasted)

- 2 tablespoons almond butter

- 1/2 cup fresh blueberries

- Honey or maple syrup for drizzling (optional)

Instructions:

1. Toast the whole grain bread slices until golden brown.

2. Spread almond butter evenly onto the toasted bread slices. Top the almond butter with fresh blueberries.

3. Optionally, drizzle honey or maple syrup over the berries for added sweetness.

Salmon and Avocado Breakfast Toast

Ingredients:

• 2 slices whole grain bread (toasted)

• 4 ounces smoked salmon

• 1 ripe avocado

• Lemon juice

• Fresh dill or parsley for garnish

• Salt and pepper to taste

Instructions:

1. Toast the whole grain bread slices until golden brown.

2. Mash the ripe avocado in a bowl and season with lemon juice, salt, and pepper.

3. Spread the mashed avocado onto the toasted bread slices. Layer smoked salmon on top of the avocado.

4. Garnish with fresh dill or parsley before serving.

Greek Yogurt Breakfast Bowl with Nuts and Berries

Ingredients:

• 1 cup Greek yogurt

• 1/4 cup mixed nuts (almonds, walnuts)

• 1/2 cup mixed berries (blueberries, raspberries)

• 1 tablespoon honey or maple syrup

• Optional: Chia seeds or shredded coconut for topping

Instructions:

1. Spoon Greek yogurt into a bowl.

2. Top the yogurt with mixed nuts and berries. Drizzle honey or maple syrup over the toppings.

3. Optionally, sprinkle chia seeds or shredded coconut for added texture and nutrients before serving.

Quinoa Breakfast Bowl with Fruits and Nuts

Ingredients:

- 1/2 cup cooked quinoa

- 1/4 cup almond milk (or any preferred milk)

- 1/2 banana (sliced)

- 1/4 cup mixed berries (blueberries, strawberries)

- 2 tablespoons chopped almonds or walnuts

- 1 tablespoon honey or maple syrup

Instructions:

1. In a bowl, mix cooked quinoa with almond milk.

2. Top the quinoa with sliced banana, mixed berries, and chopped nuts.

3. Drizzle honey or maple syrup over the bowl and enjoy.

Veggie and Egg Breakfast Skillet

Ingredients:

• 4 eggs

• 1 cup diced bell peppers (mixed colors)

• 1/2 cup diced onion

• 1 cup chopped spinach

• 2 cloves garlic (minced)

• 1 tablespoon olive oil

• Salt, pepper, and herbs of choice (optional)

Instructions:

1. Heat olive oil in a skillet over medium heat.

2. Sauté diced onions, bell peppers, and minced garlic until softened. Add chopped spinach and cook until wilted.

3. Create wells in the vegetable mixture and crack an egg into each well.

4. Season eggs with salt, pepper, and herbs if desired. Cover and cook until the eggs are done to your liking.

5. Divide the skillet into servings and serve directly from the pan.

Chia Seed and Mixed Berry Smoothie

Ingredients:

• 1 cup mixed berries (strawberries, raspberries, blueberries)

• 1 tablespoon chia seeds

• 1/2 cup Greek yogurt

• 1/2 cup almond milk (or any preferred milk)

• 1 tablespoon honey or maple syrup (optional)

Instructions:

1. In a blender, combine mixed berries, chia seeds, Greek yogurt, and almond milk.

2. Optionally, add honey or maple syrup for sweetness.

3. Blend the ingredients until you achieve a smooth consistency. Pour the smoothie into glasses and enjoy immediately.

Oatmeal with Almond Butter and Banana

Ingredients:

• 1/2 cup rolled oats

• 1 cup water or milk of choice

• 1 tablespoon almond butter

• 1/2 banana (sliced)

• Cinnamon or nutmeg for sprinkling

• Optional: Drizzle of honey or maple syrup

Instructions:

1. In a saucepan, bring water or milk to a boil.

2. Stir in rolled oats and cook according to package instructions.

3. Once cooked, transfer the oatmeal to a bowl. Top with almond butter, sliced banana, and a sprinkle of cinnamon or nutmeg.

4. Optionally, drizzle honey or maple syrup for added sweetness.

Tomato Avocado Breakfast Toast

Ingredients:

• 2 slices whole grain bread (toasted)

• 1 ripe avocado

• 1 medium tomato (sliced)

• Fresh basil leaves for garnish

• Olive oil for drizzling

• Salt and pepper to taste

Instructions:

1. Toast the whole grain bread slices until golden brown.

2. Mash the ripe avocado in a bowl and season with salt and pepper.

3. Spread the mashed avocado onto the toasted bread slices. Layer sliced tomatoes on top of the avocado.

4. Garnish with fresh basil leaves and drizzle with olive oil before serving.

Mediterranean Chickpea Salad

Ingredients:

- 1 can (15 oz) chickpeas (drained and rinsed)

- 1 cup cherry tomatoes (halved)

- 1 cucumber (diced)

- 1/4 cup red onion (finely chopped)

- 1/4 cup Kalamata olives (pitted and sliced)

- 2 tablespoons chopped fresh parsley

- 2 tablespoons olive oil

- 1 tablespoon red wine vinegar

- Salt and pepper to taste

- Crumbled feta cheese (optional)

Instructions:

1. Rinse and drain the chickpeas.

2. Halve the cherry tomatoes, dice the cucumber, chop the red onion, slice the olives, and chop the parsley.

3. In a large bowl, combine chickpeas, cherry tomatoes, cucumber, red onion, Kalamata olives, and chopped parsley.

4. Drizzle olive oil and red wine vinegar over the salad.

5. Season with salt and pepper to taste and toss until well combined.

6. If desired, sprinkle crumbled feta cheese on top before serving.

Grilled Salmon with Quinoa and Steamed Broccoli

Ingredients:

• 2 salmon fillets

• 1 cup quinoa

• 2 cups water or vegetable broth

• 2 cups broccoli florets

• Olive oil

• Lemon wedges

• Salt, pepper, and herbs (optional) for seasoning

Instructions:

1. Rinse quinoa under cold water and cook according to package instructions using water or vegetable broth.

2. Steam broccoli until tender but still crisp.

3. Preheat the grill or grill pan over medium-high heat.

4. Season salmon fillets with salt, pepper, and herbs if desired. Brush with olive oil.

5. Grill salmon for about 4-5 minutes per side or until cooked through.

6. Divide cooked quinoa, grilled salmon, and steamed broccoli onto plates. Squeeze fresh lemon juice over the salmon before serving.

Veggie and Hummus Wrap

Ingredients:

• Whole grain wraps or tortillas

• 1 cup hummus

• 1 cup mixed salad greens

• 1 bell pepper (sliced)

- 1 cucumber (sliced)

- 1/2 cup shredded carrots

- 1/4 cup red onion (sliced)

- Optional: Feta cheese or avocado slices

Instructions:

1. Lay out the whole grain wraps or tortillas.

2. Spread a layer of hummus onto each wrap.

3. Layer mixed salad greens, sliced bell pepper, cucumber, shredded carrots, and red onion on top of the hummus.

4. If desired, add crumbled feta cheese or avocado slices.

5. Roll up the wraps, folding in the sides, and serve immediately or wrap in foil for a portable lunch.

Quinoa Stuffed Bell Peppers

Ingredients:

- 4 bell peppers (any color)

- 1 cup cooked quinoa

- 1 can (15 oz) black beans (drained and rinsed)

- 1 cup corn kernels

- 1 cup diced tomatoes

- 1/2 cup diced onion

- 2 cloves garlic (minced)

- 1 teaspoon cumin

- 1 teaspoon chili powder

- Salt and pepper to taste

- Shredded cheese (optional)

Instructions:

1. Preheat the oven to 375°F (190°C).

2. Cut the tops off the bell peppers and remove the seeds and membranes.

3. In a skillet, sauté diced onions and minced garlic until translucent.

4. Add cooked quinoa, black beans, corn kernels, diced tomatoes, cumin, chili powder, salt, and pepper. Stir to combine.

5. Spoon the quinoa mixture into the hollowed-out bell peppers.

6. Optional: Sprinkle shredded cheese on top of each stuffed pepper.

7. Place the stuffed bell peppers in a baking dish and bake for 25-30 minutes or until the peppers are tender.

Lentil and Vegetable Soup

Ingredients:

• 1 cup dried lentils (rinsed and drained)

• 4 cups vegetable broth

• 1 onion (chopped)

• 2 carrots (sliced)

• 2 celery stalks (chopped)

• 2 cloves garlic (minced)

• 1 can (14 oz) diced tomatoes

• 1 teaspoon dried thyme

• 1 teaspoon dried oregano

• Salt and pepper to taste

• Fresh parsley for garnish (optional)

Instructions:

1. In a large pot, sauté chopped onions, carrots, celery, and minced garlic until softened.

2. Add dried lentils, vegetable broth, diced tomatoes, dried thyme, dried oregano, salt, and pepper to the pot. Bring to a boil.

3. Reduce heat to low, cover, and simmer for about 25-30 minutes or until the lentils are tender.

4. Ladle the lentil and vegetable soup into bowls.

5. Garnish with fresh parsley if desired before serving.

Quinoa and Black Bean Salad

Ingredients:

• 1 cup cooked quinoa

• 1 can (15 oz) black beans (drained and rinsed)

• 1 cup diced bell peppers (mixed colors)

• 1/2 cup cherry tomatoes (halved)

• 1/4 cup diced red onion

• 2 tablespoons chopped fresh cilantro or parsley

- 2 tablespoons lime juice

- 2 tablespoons olive oil

- Salt and pepper to taste

- Avocado slices (optional)

Instructions:

1. In a large bowl, mix together cooked quinoa, black beans, diced bell peppers, cherry tomatoes, diced red onion, and chopped cilantro or parsley.

2. In a separate small bowl, whisk together lime juice, olive oil, salt, and pepper.

3. Drizzle the dressing over the quinoa and bean mixture. Toss to coat evenly.

4. Optionally, add avocado slices on top before serving.

Tuna Salad Lettuce Wraps

Ingredients:

- 2 cans (5 oz each) tuna in water (drained)

- 1/4 cup diced celery

- 1/4 cup diced red onion

- 2 tablespoons chopped fresh parsley

- 2 tablespoons Greek yogurt

- 1 tablespoon lemon juice

- Salt and pepper to taste

- Lettuce leaves for wrapping

Instructions:

1. In a bowl, mix together drained tuna, diced celery, diced red onion, chopped parsley, Greek yogurt, lemon juice, salt, and pepper.

2. Spoon the tuna salad mixture onto lettuce leaves.

3. Roll up the lettuce leaves, enclosing the filling. Serve immediately.

Grilled Chicken and Vegetable Skewers

Ingredients:

- 2 boneless, skinless chicken breasts (cut into cubes)

- 1 bell pepper (cut into chunks)

- 1 zucchini (sliced)

- 1 red onion (cut into chunks)

- 8 cherry tomatoes

- 2 tablespoons olive oil

- 2 cloves garlic (minced)

- 1 teaspoon dried oregano

- Salt and pepper to taste

- Wooden skewers (pre-soaked in water)

Instructions:

1. In a bowl, combine olive oil, minced garlic, dried oregano, salt, and pepper.

2. Thread chicken cubes, bell pepper, zucchini slices, red onion chunks, and cherry tomatoes onto the wooden skewers.

3. Brush the marinade onto the skewered ingredients.

4. Preheat the grill or grill pan over medium-high heat.

5. Grill the skewers for about 10-12 minutes, turning occasionally, until chicken is cooked through and vegetables are slightly charred.

6. Remove skewers from the grill and serve immediately.

Eggplant and Tomato Pasta

Ingredients:

• 8 oz whole grain pasta (such as penne or spaghetti)

• 1 large eggplant (cubed)

• 2 cups diced tomatoes

• 3 cloves garlic (minced)

• 2 tablespoons olive oil

• 1/4 cup chopped fresh basil

• Salt and pepper to taste

• Grated Parmesan cheese (optional)

Instructions:

1. Cook the whole grain pasta according to package instructions. Drain and set aside.

2. Heat olive oil in a skillet over medium heat.

3. Add minced garlic and cubed eggplant. Cook until eggplant softens.

4. Stir in diced tomatoes and cook until heated through.

5. Add the cooked pasta to the skillet with the eggplant and tomatoes. Toss to combine and coat the pasta with the vegetable mixture.

6. Season with salt, pepper, and chopped fresh basil. Optionally, sprinkle with grated Parmesan cheese before serving.

Spinach and Chickpea Curry

Ingredients:

• 1 can (15 oz) chickpeas (drained and rinsed)

• 2 cups fresh spinach leaves

• 1 onion (chopped)

• 2 tomatoes (chopped)

• 3 cloves garlic (minced)

• 1 teaspoon grated ginger

• 1 teaspoon ground cumin

• 1 teaspoon ground coriander

• 1/2 teaspoon turmeric

• 1/2 teaspoon paprika

- 1/4 teaspoon cayenne pepper (optional for heat)

- 1 cup vegetable broth

- 2 tablespoons olive oil

- Salt and pepper to taste

- Cooked brown rice or whole grain bread for serving

Instructions:

1. Heat olive oil in a large skillet over medium heat.

2. Sauté chopped onion until translucent, then add minced garlic and grated ginger. Cook until fragrant.

3. Add ground cumin, ground coriander, turmeric, paprika, and cayenne pepper. Stir for a minute.

4. Add chopped tomatoes to the skillet and cook until they break down. Stir in chickpeas and vegetable broth. Simmer for 5-7 minutes.

5. Add fresh spinach leaves to the skillet and cook until wilted.

6. Season with salt and pepper to taste.

7. Serve the spinach and chickpea curry with cooked brown rice or whole grain bread.

Veggie Quinoa Bowl with Lemon-Tahini Dressing

Ingredients:

• 1 cup cooked quinoa

• 1 cup mixed vegetables (such as roasted carrots, bell peppers, and steamed broccoli)

• 1/4 cup chickpeas (cooked or canned)

• 2 tablespoons chopped fresh parsley

Lemon-Tahini Dressing:

• 2 tablespoons tahini

• 2 tablespoons fresh lemon juice

• 1 tablespoon olive oil

• 1 clove garlic (minced)

• Salt and pepper to taste

• Water (to thin if necessary)

Instructions:

1. Cook quinoa according to package instructions.

2. Roast or steam mixed vegetables until tender.

3. In a bowl, combine cooked quinoa, mixed vegetables, chickpeas, and chopped parsley.

4. In a small bowl, whisk together tahini, lemon juice, olive oil, minced garlic, salt, and pepper. If too thick, add water gradually to reach desired consistency.

5. Drizzle the lemon-tahini dressing over the quinoa bowl before serving.

Turkey and Avocado Wrap

Ingredients:

• Whole grain wraps or tortillas

• Sliced turkey breast

• 1 avocado (sliced)

• 1/4 cup shredded lettuce or mixed greens

• 2 tablespoons Greek yogurt or hummus

• 1 tablespoon Dijon mustard

• Salt and pepper to taste

Instructions:

1. Lay out the whole grain wraps or tortillas.

2. Spread Greek yogurt or hummus onto each wrap.

3. Layer sliced turkey, avocado, shredded lettuce or mixed greens on top. Season with Dijon mustard, salt, and pepper.

4. Roll up the wraps, folding in the sides, and serve immediately or pack for a portable lunch.

Quinoa Stuffed Bell Pepper Soup

Ingredients:

• 1 cup cooked quinoa

• 4 bell peppers (any color)

• 1 can (15 oz) diced tomatoes

• 2 cups vegetable broth

• 1 onion (diced)

• 2 cloves garlic (minced)

• 1 teaspoon dried basil

• 1 teaspoon dried oregano

• 1/2 teaspoon paprika

• Salt and pepper to taste

• Olive oil for cooking

Instructions:

1. Cut the tops off the bell peppers, remove seeds, and chop the edible parts.

2. In a pot, heat olive oil over medium heat. Sauté diced onion and minced garlic until softened.

3. Add chopped bell peppers, diced tomatoes, cooked quinoa, vegetable broth, dried basil, dried oregano, paprika, salt, and pepper to the pot.

4. Bring to a boil, then reduce heat and simmer for about 20-25 minutes.

5. Ladle the quinoa-stuffed bell pepper soup into bowls and serve hot.

Lentil and Vegetable Stir-Fry

Ingredients:

• 1 cup cooked lentils

• 2 cups mixed vegetables (such as broccoli, bell peppers, snap peas)

• 2 tablespoons low-sodium soy sauce or tamari

- 1 tablespoon sesame oil

- 2 cloves garlic (minced)

- 1 teaspoon grated ginger

- Sesame seeds for garnish

- Cooked brown rice for serving

Instructions:

1. Cook lentils according to package instructions. Chop vegetables into bite-sized pieces.

2. Heat sesame oil in a skillet or wok over medium-high heat.

3. Sauté minced garlic and grated ginger until fragrant. Add mixed vegetables and stir-fry until they start to soften.

4. Add cooked lentils and low-sodium soy sauce (or tamari) to the skillet. Stir well to combine and cook for an additional 2-3 minutes.

5. Serve the lentil and vegetable stir-fry over cooked brown rice, garnished with sesame seeds.

Spinach and Tomato Frittata

Ingredients:

• 6 eggs

• 1 cup fresh spinach leaves

• 1 tomato (sliced)

• 1/2 onion (chopped)

• 1/4 cup shredded cheese (optional)

• 2 tablespoons olive oil

• Salt and pepper to taste

Instructions:

1. Preheat the oven to 350°F (175°C).

2. In an ovenproof skillet, heat olive oil over medium heat.

3. Sauté chopped onion until translucent, then add fresh spinach and cook until wilted.

4. In a bowl, whisk eggs and season with salt and pepper. Pour the whisked eggs into the skillet over the sautéed vegetables.

5. Place tomato slices on top of the egg mixture. Optionally, sprinkle shredded cheese on top.

6. Transfer the skillet to the preheated oven and bake for about 15-20 minutes or until the frittata is set in the center.

7. Slice the spinach and tomato frittata into wedges and serve.

Mediterranean Chickpea Wraps

Ingredients:

• Whole grain wraps or tortillas

• 1 can (15 oz) chickpeas (drained and rinsed)

• 1/2 cup diced cucumber

• 1/2 cup diced tomatoes

• 1/4 cup chopped red onion

• 2 tablespoons chopped fresh parsley

• 2 tablespoons lemon juice

• 2 tablespoons olive oil

• Salt and pepper to taste

• Optional: Hummus or tzatziki sauce

Instructions:

1. In a bowl, combine chickpeas, diced cucumber, diced tomatoes, chopped red onion, chopped parsley, lemon juice, olive oil, salt, and pepper.

2. Lay out the whole grain wraps or tortillas.

3. Spread a layer of hummus or tzatziki sauce on each wrap. Spoon the chickpea salad onto the wraps.

4. Roll up the wraps, folding in the sides, and serve immediately or wrap in foil for later.

Baked Salmon with Herb Quinoa

Ingredients:

• 2 salmon fillets

• 1 cup quinoa

• 2 cups chicken or vegetable broth

• 2 tablespoons chopped fresh dill

• 2 tablespoons chopped fresh parsley

• 1 lemon (sliced)

• Olive oil

• Salt and pepper to taste

Instructions:

1. Preheat the oven to 375°F (190°C).

2. Rinse quinoa under cold water and cook according to package instructions using chicken or vegetable broth.

3. Place salmon fillets on a baking sheet lined with parchment paper.

4. Drizzle salmon with olive oil, sprinkle with salt, pepper, chopped dill, and parsley. Place lemon slices on top of the salmon.

5. Bake in the preheated oven for about 12-15 minutes or until the salmon is cooked through.

6. Serve the baked salmon over herb quinoa.

Veggie and Brown Rice Stir-Fry

Ingredients:

• 2 cups cooked brown rice

• 2 cups mixed vegetables (such as bell peppers, broccoli, carrots)

• 1 cup snap peas

- 1/4 cup low-sodium soy sauce or tamari

- 2 cloves garlic (minced)

- 1 teaspoon grated ginger

- 2 tablespoons sesame oil

- 2 tablespoons chopped green onions

- Sesame seeds for garnish

Instructions:

1. Heat sesame oil in a large skillet or wok over medium-high heat.

2. Add minced garlic and grated ginger, sauté for a minute. Add mixed vegetables and snap peas, stir-fry until tender-crisp.

3. Add cooked brown rice to the skillet.

4. Pour low-sodium soy sauce or tamari over the rice and vegetables, toss to combine.

5. Stir in chopped green onions. Garnish with sesame seeds before serving.

Caprese Salad with Grilled Chicken

Ingredients:

• 2 boneless, skinless chicken breasts

• 2 large tomatoes (sliced)

• 1 cup fresh basil leaves

• 8 oz fresh mozzarella cheese (sliced)

• Balsamic glaze (store-bought or homemade)

• Olive oil

• Salt and pepper to taste

Instructions:

1. Preheat the grill or grill pan over medium-high heat.

2. Season chicken breasts with olive oil, salt, and pepper. Grill chicken for about 6-8 minutes per side or until cooked through.

3. On a serving platter, alternate slices of tomato, fresh basil leaves, and fresh mozzarella cheese.

4. Slice the grilled chicken breasts and place them on top of the Caprese salad.

5. Drizzle balsamic glaze over the salad and chicken before serving.

Lemon Garlic Shrimp with Quinoa

Ingredients:

• 1-pound large shrimp (peeled and deveined)

• 1 cup cooked quinoa

• 2 tablespoons olive oil

• 3 cloves garlic (minced)

• Zest and juice of 1 lemon

• 2 tablespoons chopped fresh parsley

• Salt and pepper to taste

Instructions:

1. Cook quinoa according to package instructions and set aside.

2. Heat olive oil in a skillet over medium-high heat.

3. Add minced garlic and sauté for about 30 seconds. Add shrimp to the skillet, cook for 2-3 minutes per side or until shrimp turn pink.

4. Season shrimp with lemon zest, lemon juice, chopped parsley, salt, and pepper.

5. Toss cooked quinoa with the shrimp mixture.

6. Serve the lemon garlic shrimp over quinoa.

Tofu Veggie Stir-Fry

Ingredients:

• 1 block firm tofu (pressed and cubed)

• 2 cups mixed vegetables (such as bell peppers, broccoli, carrots)

• 2 cloves garlic (minced)

• 1 tablespoon grated ginger

• 2 tablespoons low-sodium soy sauce or tamari

• 1 tablespoon sesame oil

• 2 tablespoons chopped green onions

• 1 tablespoon sesame seeds

• Cooked brown rice or quinoa for serving

Instructions:

1. Press tofu to remove excess water, then cut into cubes.

2. Heat sesame oil in a skillet or wok over medium-high heat. Sauté tofu cubes until golden brown. Remove and set aside.

3. In the same skillet, sauté minced garlic and grated ginger until fragrant. Add mixed vegetables and stir-fry until tender-crisp.

4. Return the cooked tofu to the skillet with the vegetables. Add low-sodium soy sauce or tamari. Stir well to combine.

5. Garnish with chopped green onions and sesame seeds.

6. Serve over cooked brown rice or quinoa.

Chicken and Vegetable Kebabs

Ingredients:

• 2 boneless, skinless chicken breasts (cut into chunks)

• 1 red bell pepper (cut into chunks)

• 1 yellow bell pepper (cut into chunks)

• 1 red onion (cut into chunks)

• 8-10 cherry tomatoes

• 2 tablespoons olive oil

• 2 cloves garlic (minced)

- 1 teaspoon dried oregano

- 1 teaspoon paprika

- Salt and pepper to taste

- Wooden skewers (pre-soaked in water)

Instructions:

1. In a bowl, mix olive oil, minced garlic, dried oregano, paprika, salt, and pepper.

2. Thread chicken chunks, bell peppers, red onion chunks, and cherry tomatoes onto the skewers.

3. Brush the marinade onto the skewered ingredients.

4. Preheat the grill or grill pan over medium-high heat.

5. Grill the skewers for about 10-12 minutes, turning occasionally, until chicken is cooked through and vegetables are slightly charred.

6. Remove skewers from the grill and serve immediately.

Ingredients:

• 1 prepared whole grain pie crust

• 6 large eggs

• 1 cup fresh spinach (chopped)

• 1 cup sliced mushrooms

• 1/2 cup diced onion

• 1 cup shredded cheese (such as Gruyère or Swiss)

• 1 cup milk or unsweetened almond milk

• Salt and pepper to taste

• Olive oil

Instructions:

1. Preheat the oven to 375°F (190°C).

2. In a skillet, heat olive oil over medium heat.

3. Sauté diced onion until translucent, then add sliced mushrooms and chopped spinach. Cook until vegetables soften.

4. Remove from heat and let cool.

5. In a bowl, whisk together eggs, milk, shredded cheese, salt, and pepper.

6. Spread the sautéed vegetable mixture evenly into the prepared pie crust. Pour the egg and cheese mixture over the vegetables.

7. Place the quiche in the preheated oven and bake for about 35-40 minutes or until the center is set and the crust is golden brown.

8. Allow the quiche to cool slightly before slicing and serving.

Tomato Basil Pasta Salad

Ingredients:

• 8 oz whole grain pasta (such as penne or fusilli)

• 2 cups cherry tomatoes (halved)

• 1/4 cup chopped fresh basil

• 1/4 cup sliced black olives

• 2 tablespoons olive oil

• 2 tablespoons balsamic vinegar

• 2 cloves garlic (minced)

- Salt and pepper to taste

- Optional: Feta cheese crumbles

Instructions:

1. Cook the whole grain pasta according to package instructions. Drain and set aside to cool.

2. In a small bowl, whisk together olive oil, balsamic vinegar, minced garlic, salt, and pepper.

3. In a large bowl, combine cooked pasta, cherry tomatoes, chopped basil, sliced black olives, and the prepared dressing. Toss gently to combine.

4. If desired, sprinkle feta cheese crumbles over the pasta salad.

5. Refrigerate the pasta salad for at least 30 minutes before serving.

Broccoli and Almond Soup

Ingredients:

- 2 cups broccoli florets

- 1/2 cup almonds (toasted)

- 1 onion (chopped)

- 2 cloves garlic (minced)

- 4 cups vegetable broth

- 1 tablespoon olive oil

- Salt and pepper to taste

Instructions:

1. In a pot, heat olive oil over medium heat. Sauté chopped onion and minced garlic until softened.

2. Add broccoli florets to the pot and cook for a few minutes.

3. Pour in vegetable broth and bring to a boil. Simmer for about 15-20 minutes until broccoli is tender.

4. Using an immersion blender or transferring to a blender, blend the soup until smooth.

5. Stir in toasted almonds (reserving some for garnish), and season with salt and pepper to taste.

6. Ladle the broccoli and almond soup into bowls and garnish with remaining toasted almonds before serving.

Lemon Herb Chicken with Roasted Vegetables

Ingredients:

• 2 boneless, skinless chicken breasts

• 2 cups mixed vegetables (such as carrots, bell peppers, zucchini)

• 2 tablespoons olive oil

• 2 cloves garlic (minced)

• 1 tablespoon fresh thyme (chopped)

• Zest and juice of 1 lemon

• Salt and pepper to taste

Instructions:

1. Preheat the oven to 400°F (200°C).

2. Place chicken breasts and mixed vegetables on a baking sheet. Drizzle olive oil over the chicken and vegetables.

3. Sprinkle minced garlic, chopped thyme, lemon zest, lemon juice, salt, and pepper over everything.

4. Bake in the preheated oven for about 20-25 minutes or until the chicken is cooked through and vegetables are tender.

5. Serve the lemon herb chicken with roasted vegetables.

Quinoa and Black Bean Stuffed Bell Peppers

Ingredients:

• 4 bell peppers (any color)

• 1 cup cooked quinoa

• 1 can (15 oz) black beans (drained and rinsed)

• 1 cup corn kernels

• 1 cup diced tomatoes

• 1/2 cup diced onion

• 2 cloves garlic (minced)

• 1 teaspoon cumin

• 1 teaspoon chili powder

• Salt and pepper to taste

• Shredded cheese (optional)

Instructions:

1. Preheat the oven to 375°F (190°C).

2. Cut the tops off the bell peppers, remove seeds, and set aside.

3. In a skillet, sauté diced onions and minced garlic until translucent.

4. Add cooked quinoa, black beans, corn kernels, diced tomatoes, cumin, chili powder, salt, and pepper. Stir to combine.

5. Spoon the quinoa mixture into the hollowed-out bell peppers. Optionally, sprinkle shredded cheese on top of each stuffed pepper.

6. Place the stuffed bell peppers in a baking dish and bake for 25-30 minutes or until the peppers are tender.

Asian-style Tofu and Broccoli Stir-Fry

Ingredients:

• 1 block firm tofu (pressed and cubed)

• 2 cups broccoli florets

• 1 bell pepper (sliced)

• 2 cloves garlic (minced)

• 1 tablespoon grated ginger

• 3 tablespoons low-sodium soy sauce or tamari

• 1 tablespoon rice vinegar

- 1 tablespoon honey or maple syrup

- 2 tablespoons sesame oil

- Cooked brown rice for serving

Instructions:

1. Heat sesame oil in a skillet or wok over medium-high heat.

2. Sauté cubed tofu until golden brown. Remove and set aside.

3. In the same skillet, stir-fry minced garlic, grated ginger, broccoli florets, and sliced bell pepper until tender-crisp.

4. In a small bowl, mix low-sodium soy sauce or tamari, rice vinegar, and honey or maple syrup.

5. Return the cooked tofu to the skillet with the vegetables.

6. Pour the sauce over the tofu and vegetables. Stir well to coat evenly.

7. Serve the tofu and broccoli stir-fry over cooked brown rice.

Mediterranean Chickpea Salad with Couscous

Ingredients:

• 1 cup cooked couscous

• 1 can (15 oz) chickpeas (drained and rinsed)

• 1 cup cherry tomatoes (halved)

• 1 cucumber (diced)

• 1/4 cup red onion (finely chopped)

• 1/4 cup Kalamata olives (pitted and sliced)

• 2 tablespoons chopped fresh parsley

• 2 tablespoons olive oil

• 1 tablespoon red wine vinegar

• Salt and pepper to taste

• Crumbled feta cheese (optional)

Instructions:

1. Cook couscous according to package instructions. Rinse and drain the chickpeas.

2. Halve the cherry tomatoes, dice the cucumber, chop the red onion, slice the olives, and chop the parsley.

3. In a large bowl, combine cooked couscous, chickpeas, cherry tomatoes, cucumber, red onion, Kalamata olives, and chopped parsley.

4. Drizzle olive oil and red wine vinegar over the salad. Season with salt and pepper to taste and toss until well combined.

5. If desired, sprinkle crumbled feta cheese on top before serving.

Veggie Frittata with Spinach and Bell Peppers

Ingredients:

• 6 eggs

• 1 cup fresh spinach (chopped)

• 1 bell pepper (diced)

• 1/2 cup diced onion

• 1/2 cup shredded cheese (such as cheddar or mozzarella)

• 2 tablespoons olive oil

• Salt and pepper to taste

Instructions:

1. Preheat the oven to 350°F (175°C).

2. In an ovenproof skillet, heat olive oil over medium heat.

3. Sauté diced onion until translucent, then add diced bell pepper and cook until softened.

4. Add chopped spinach and cook until wilted. Spread the vegetables evenly in the skillet.

5. In a bowl, whisk eggs and season with salt and pepper. Pour the whisked eggs over the sautéed vegetables in the skillet.

6. Sprinkle shredded cheese evenly over the egg mixture.

7. Transfer the skillet to the preheated oven and bake for about 20-25 minutes or until the frittata is set in the center.

8. Allow the frittata to cool slightly, then slice and serve.

Walnut-Rosemary Crusted Salmon

Ingredients:

• 2 teaspoons Dijon mustard

• 1 clove garlic, minced

• ¼ teaspoon lemon zest

• 1 teaspoon lemon juice

• 1 teaspoon chopped fresh rosemary

• ½ teaspoon honey

• ½ teaspoon kosher salt

• ¼ teaspoon crushed red pepper

• 3 tablespoons panko breadcrumbs

• 3 tablespoons finely chopped walnuts

• 1 teaspoon extra-virgin olive oil

• 1 (1 pound) skinless salmon fillet, fresh or frozen

• Olive oil cooking spray

• Chopped fresh parsley and lemon wedges for garnish

Instructions:

1. Preheat oven to 425 degrees F. Line a large rimmed baking sheet with parchment paper.

2. Combine mustard, garlic, lemon zest, lemon juice, rosemary, honey, salt and crushed red pepper in a small bowl. Combine panko, walnuts and oil in another small bowl.

3. Place salmon on the prepared baking sheet. Spread the mustard mixture over the fish and sprinkle with the panko mixture, pressing to adhere. Lightly coat with cooking spray.

4. Bake until the fish flakes easily with a fork, about 8 to 12 minutes, depending on thickness.

5. Sprinkle with parsley and serve with lemon wedges, if desired.

Easy Fish Tacos with Kiwi Salsa

Ingredients:

• 1 cup thinly sliced red cabbage

• 1 tablespoon rice vinegar

• 1 cup diced peeled kiwi

• 2 tablespoons finely diced red onion

- 1 tablespoon chopped fresh cilantro

- 1 tablespoon lime juice

- 1 teaspoon finely chopped jalapeño pepper, plus slices for garnish

- ¾ cup white whole-wheat flour, divided

- 1 teaspoon baking powder

- ¼ teaspoon salt plus a pinch, divided

- ½ cup Mexican lager

- 8 ounces skinned center-cut firm white fish, such as cod

- 2 cups corn oil

- 8 corn tortillas, warmed

Instructions:

1. Toss cabbage with vinegar in a medium bowl. Combine kiwi, onion, cilantro, lime juice and jalapeño in a small bowl. Set aside.

2. Whisk 1/2 cup flour, baking powder, 1/4 teaspoon salt and beer in a medium bowl. Cut fish into 8 pieces. Dust with the remaining 1/4 cup flour. Shake off the excess flour and add the fish to the batter, turning to coat.

3. Place a wire rack on a baking sheet near the stove. Heat oil in a medium skillet over medium-high heat to 325 degrees F. Let excess batter drip off, then add half the fish to the pan. Cook, turning once, until the coating is golden, about 3 minutes total. Transfer to the rack, let the oil heat back to 325 degrees F and repeat with the remaining fish. Sprinkle with the remaining pinch of salt.

4. Serve the fish in tortillas with the reserved cabbage, kiwi salsa and jalapeño slices, if desired.

Crispy Chickpea Grain Bowl with Lemon Vinaigrette

Ingredients:

• ⅔ cup quinoa

• 1 ⅓ cups water plus 1 tablespoon, divided

• ⅛ teaspoon salt plus 1/4 teaspoon, divided

• 1 (15 ounce) can no-salt-added chickpeas, rinsed

• 1 small red onion, thinly sliced

• 4 teaspoons extra-virgin olive oil plus 2 tablespoons, divided

• ¼ teaspoon ground pepper, divided

• 1 bunch kale, stems removed, thinly sliced (about 5 cups)

- 1 teaspoon Dijon mustard

- 1 clove garlic, minced

- 2 teaspoons lemon zest

- 2 tablespoons lemon juice

- 1 red bell pepper, thinly sliced

- ¼ cup crumbled feta cheese

- 2 tablespoons toasted pumpkin seeds

Instructions:

1. Preheat oven to 400 degrees F. Coat a large rimmed baking sheet liberally with cooking spray.

2. Combine quinoa, 1 1/3 cups water, and 1/8 teaspoon salt in a medium saucepan. Bring to a boil over medium-high heat. Reduce heat to medium-low, partially cover, and simmer until the quinoa is tender, about 15 minutes. Drain any excess water.

3. Meanwhile, pat chickpeas dry with a paper towel. Toss with onion, 2 teaspoons oil, and 1/8 teaspoon each salt and pepper in a large bowl. Spread out on the prepared baking sheet. Roast for 15 minutes.

4. Toss kale with 2 teaspoons oil and the remaining 1/8 teaspoon salt in the large bowl. Stir the kale into the chickpeas and roast for 15 minutes more.

5. Whisk mustard, garlic, lemon zest, lemon juice, the remaining 1 tablespoon water and the remaining 1/8 teaspoon pepper in a small bowl. Whisk in the remaining 2 tablespoons oil.

6. Divide the quinoa among 4 serving bowls. Top with the kale mixture, bell pepper slices, feta, and pumpkin seeds. Drizzle with the vinaigrette.

Grilled Lemon-Pepper Salmon in Foil

Ingredients:

• 4 (6 ounce) skin-on salmon fillets

• 2 tablespoons unsalted butter

• 1 teaspoon lemon pepper

• ½ teaspoon salt

• 8 thin slices lemon (from 1 lemon)

• 4 sprigs flat-leaf parsley

Instructions:

1. Preheat grill to medium-high (400-450 degrees F). Place 4 (12-inch) foil squares in a single layer on a work surface; coat with cooking spray.

2. Place 1 salmon fillet, skin-side down, in the center of each. Top each fillet with 1 1/2 teaspoons butter, 1/4 teaspoon lemon pepper, 1/8 teaspoon salt, 2 lemon slices and 1 parsley sprig. Crimp the sides of each foil packet together to tightly seal.

3. Place the packets on the grill; cover and grill until the fish flakes easily with a fork, 8 to 10 minutes.

White Bean and Sun-Dried Tomato Gnocchi

Ingredients:

• ½ cup sliced oil-packed sun-dried tomatoes plus 2 tablespoons oil from the jar, divided

• 1 (16 ounce) package shelf-stable gnocchi

• 1 (15 ounce) can low-sodium cannellini beans, rinsed

• 1 (5 ounce) package baby spinach

• 1 large shallot, minced

• ⅓ cup low-sodium no-chicken broth or chicken broth

• ⅓ cup heavy cream

• 1 tablespoon lemon juice

• ¼ teaspoon salt

- ¼ teaspoon ground pepper

- 3 tablespoons fresh basil leaves

Instructions:

1. Heat 1 tablespoon oil in a large nonstick skillet over medium-high heat.

2. Add gnocchi and cook, stirring often, until plumped and starting to brown, about 5 minutes. Add beans and spinach and cook until the spinach is wilted, about 1 minute. Transfer to a plate.

3. Add the remaining 1 tablespoon oil to the pan and heat over medium heat. Add sun-dried tomatoes and shallot; cook, stirring, for 1 minute. Increase heat to high and add broth. Cook until the liquid has mostly evaporated, about 2 minutes.

4. Reduce heat to medium and stir in cream, lemon juice, salt and pepper. Return the gnocchi mixture to the pan and stir to coat with the sauce. Serve topped with basil.

Tofu and Roasted Vegetable Grain Bowl with Pumpkin Seeds

Ingredients:

- 8 ounces extra-firm tofu, cut into 1-inch cubes

- 5 tablespoons plus 1 teaspoon extra-virgin olive oil, divided

- 1 tablespoon reduced-sodium tamari or soy sauce

- ½ teaspoon chili powder

- 1 medium red bell pepper, cut into 1/2-inch strips

- ½ medium red onion, cut into 1/2-inch wedges

- ½ avocado

- ⅓ cup water

- ¼ cup packed cilantro leaves, plus more for garnish

- 2 tablespoons lime juice

- ½ teaspoon ground coriander

- ¼ teaspoon salt

- 1 cup cooked brown rice

- ½ cup chopped romaine lettuce

- 6 cherry tomatoes, halved

- 2 tablespoons toasted pumpkin seeds

Instructions:

1. Preheat oven to 425 degrees F. Line a rimmed baking sheet with parchment paper.

2. Toss tofu, 1 tablespoon oil, tamari (or soy sauce) and chili powder in a medium bowl. Place on one side of the prepared baking sheet. Add pepper, onion and 1 teaspoon oil to the bowl; stir to coat.

3. Place the vegetables on the other side of the baking sheet. Roast until the vegetables are tender and the tofu is sizzling, about 20 minutes.

4. Meanwhile, combine the remaining 4 tablespoons oil, avocado, water, cilantro, lime juice, coriander and salt in a blender jar or mini food processor. Process until smooth, scraping the sides down as necessary.

5. Place 1/2 cup rice in each of 2 shallow serving bowls. Top with the tofu, roasted vegetables, lettuce and tomatoes. Spoon 4 tablespoons dressing over each bowl and sprinkle with pumpkin seeds.

Roasted Salmon Rice Bowl with Beets and Brussels

Ingredients:

• 1 cup wild rice blend

• 2 medium golden beets, peeled and cut into 1/2-inch wedges

• 8 ounces Brussels sprouts, trimmed and halved

• 3 tablespoons extra-virgin olive oil, divided

- ¾ teaspoon salt, divided

- ¾ teaspoon ground pepper, divided

- 1 lemon

- 1 pound wild-caught salmon fillet, cut into 4 portions

- 2 rosemary sprigs, cut in half

- 2 tablespoons chopped fresh herbs, such as thyme, basil or rosemary

- 1 clove garlic, minced

- 1 tablespoon chopped pistachios

Instructions:

1. Preheat oven to 425 degrees F.

2. Cook rice blend according to package directions.

3. Meanwhile, toss beets and Brussels sprouts with 1 tablespoon oil and 1/4 teaspoon each salt and pepper in a medium bowl.

4. After the rice has cooked for 10 minutes, spread the vegetables on a large rimmed baking sheet and roast until just beginning to brown and soften, about 15 minutes.

5. Cut lemon in half crosswise. Cut half the lemon into 4 slices (reserve the other lemon half). Push the beets and Brussels sprouts to one side of the baking sheet and place salmon on the empty half.

6. Sprinkle the salmon with 1/4 teaspoon each salt and pepper and top each piece of salmon with a rosemary sprig and a lemon slice. Continue roasting until the vegetables have softened and the salmon is opaque in the center, 9 to 11 minutes more.

7. Meanwhile, squeeze the juice from the remaining lemon half into a small bowl. Whisk in the remaining 2 tablespoons oil, herbs, garlic and the remaining 1/4 teaspoon each salt and pepper.

8. Divide the rice among 4 bowls. Discard the lemon slices and rosemary sprig. Arrange the salmon and vegetables on top of the rice. Drizzle each serving with about 1 tablespoon lemon juice mixture and sprinkle with pistachios.

Herby Fish with Wilted Greens and Mushrooms

Ingredients:

- 3 tablespoons olive oil, divided

- ½ large sweet onion, sliced

- 3 cups sliced cremini mushrooms

- 2 cloves garlic, sliced

- 4 cups chopped kale

- 1 medium tomato, diced

- 2 teaspoons Mediterranean Herb Mix, divided

- 1 tablespoon lemon juice

- ½ teaspoon salt, divided

- ½ teaspoon ground pepper, divided

- 4 (4 ounce) cod, sole, or tilapia fillets

- Chopped fresh parsley, for garnish

Instructions:

1. Heat 1 Tbsp. oil in a large saucepan over medium heat. Add onion; cook, stirring occasionally, until translucent, 3 to 4 minutes. Add mushrooms and garlic; cook, stirring occasionally, until the mushrooms release their liquid and begin to brown, 4 to 6 minutes.

2. Add kale, tomato, and 1 tsp. herb mix. Cook, stirring occasionally, until the kale is wilted and the mushrooms are tender, 5 to 7 minutes. Stir in lemon juice and 1/4 tsp. each salt and pepper. Remove from heat, cover, and keep warm.

3. Sprinkle fish with the remaining 1 tsp. herb mix and 1/4 tsp. each salt and pepper. Heat the remaining 2 Tbsp. oil in a large nonstick skillet over medium-high heat. Add the fish and cook until the flesh is opaque, 2 to 4 minutes per side, depending on thickness. Transfer the fish to 4 plates or a serving platter. Top and surround the fish with the vegetables; sprinkle with parsley, if desired.

Mediterranean Herb Mix

Ingredients:

- 2 tablespoons dried oregano

- 2 tablespoons dried rosemary

- 2 tablespoons dried thyme

- 1 tablespoon dried mint

- 1 tablespoon dried sage

Instructions:

1. Combine oregano, rosemary, thyme, mint, and sage in a clean glass jar with a tight-fitting lid. Secure the lid and shake until the seasonings are mixed well.

2. Store in a cool, dry place (or the fridge) for up to 6 months. Just before using, crush the herbs between your fingers, with a mortar and pestle, or in a spice mill to release their flavors.

Pickled Beet, Arugula and Herbed Goat Cheese Sandwich

Ingredients:

• 2 ounces goat cheese, softened

• 1 tablespoon snipped chives

• 1 tablespoon chopped fresh dill

• 1 teaspoon extra-virgin olive oil

• Pinch of salt

• Ground pepper to taste

• 2 slices whole-wheat sandwich bread, lightly toasted

• 1 tablespoon chopped walnuts, toasted

• 2 ounces sliced pickled beets

• 1 cup arugula

Instructions:

1. Mash goat cheese, chives, dill, oil, salt and pepper together in a small bowl. Spread the goat cheese mixture on one side of each toast slice.

2. Sprinkle walnuts over one slice then layer on beets and arugula. Top with the second slice of toast, cheese-side down, and cut the sandwich in half.

20-Minute Creamy Tomato Salmon Skillet

Ingredients:

• 1 ¼ pounds salmon fillet, skinned and cut into 4 portions

• ¼ teaspoon salt, divided

• ¼ teaspoon ground pepper, divided

• 2 tablespoons olive oil, divided

• 1 medium zucchini, halved lengthwise and thinly sliced

• ½ cup chopped onion

• ⅓ cup dry white wine

• 1 (15 ounce) can no-salt-added diced tomatoes

• 2 ounces cream cheese, cut into cubes

- 1 teaspoon Italian seasoning

- ½ teaspoon garlic powder

- ¼ cup chopped fresh basil

Instructions:

1. Pat salmon dry and sprinkle with 1/8 teaspoon each salt and pepper. Heat 1 tablespoon oil in a large skillet over medium-high heat.

2. Add the salmon and cook until the underside is browned and releases easily from the pan, 3 to 4 minutes. Flip the salmon and continue to cook until opaque in the center, another 2 to 3 minutes. Transfer to a plate.

3. Meanwhile, add the remaining 1 tablespoon oil, zucchini and onion to the pan. Cook, stirring, until starting to soften, about 3 minutes.

4. Increase heat to medium-high and add wine. Cook, stirring, until the liquid has mostly evaporated, about 2 minutes. Add tomatoes, cream cheese, Italian seasoning, garlic powder and the remaining 1/8 teaspoon each salt and pepper.

5. Bring to a simmer and cook, stirring, until the cream cheese is melted, 4 to 5 minutes. Return the salmon to the pan and turn to coat with the sauce. Serve topped with basil.

Ingredients:

- ½ cup rinsed no-salt-added canned white beans

- 1 large egg, lightly beaten

- 3 teaspoons Dijon mustard, divided

- 1 teaspoon lemon zest

- 1 teaspoon dried dill

- 1 teaspoon dried mint

- ½ teaspoon dried tarragon

- 2 (5 ounce) cans wild albacore tuna packed in oil, drained

- ¾ cup whole-wheat panko breadcrumbs

- 6 tablespoons extra-virgin olive oil, divided

- 3 tablespoons lemon juice

- 1 teaspoon honey

- ½ teaspoon ground pepper

- ¼ teaspoon salt

- 1 (5 ounce) package spring mix salad greens

Instructions:

1. Coarsely mash beans with a fork or potato masher in a large bowl. Stir in egg, 2 teaspoons mustard, lemon zest, dill, mint and tarragon. Flake tuna into chunks; gently fold into the bean mixture. Sprinkle panko over the mixture; gently fold in until well combined. Form the mixture into 4 (1-inch-thick) patties.

2. Heat 1 tablespoon oil in a large nonstick skillet over medium heat. Swirl to coat the pan. Cook the patties until golden brown on both sides, about 3 minutes per side.

3. Whisk lemon juice, honey, pepper, salt and the remaining 1 teaspoon mustard and 5 tablespoons oil in a small bowl. Divide greens among 4 plates; top each with a tuna cake and drizzle evenly with dressing.

Garlicky Spinach and Chickpea Soup with Lemon and Pecorino Romano

Ingredients:

• Two 15-ounce cans chickpeas

• Extra-virgin olive oil

• 1 large yellow onion, roughly chopped

• 4 or 5 large garlic cloves, minced

- Kosher salt

- 1 teaspoon ground cumin

- 1 teaspoon ground coriander

- ¾ teaspoon sweet paprika

- ½ teaspoon crushed red pepper flakes

- ½ teaspoon freshly ground black pepper

- 4 cups vegetable stock or low-sodium chicken broth

- 2 cups (packed) fresh baby spinach (2 to 3 ounces)

- ½ cup roughly chopped fresh flat-leaf parsley

- 1 large lemon, cut in half

- ½ cup grated Pecorino Romano cheese

- Crusty bread, for serving

Instructions:

1. Drain the chickpeas, reserving ½ cup of their liquid.

2. In a large pot, heat 3 tablespoons of the olive oil over medium heat until shimmering. Add the onion and garlic and season with a big pinch of salt (about ½ teaspoon). Cook over medium heat, stirring regularly, until fragrant, about 5 minutes. Add the

cumin, coriander, paprika, red pepper flakes and black pepper and cook, stirring regularly for about 30 seconds.

3. Add the chickpeas and stir to coat with the spices. Using a potato masher or the back of a sturdy fork, roughly mash the chickpeas (you're just looking to break some of them up).

4. Add the stock and the reserved chickpea liquid. Increase the heat and bring to a boil, then boil for 5 minutes. Reduce the heat to medium-low and partly cover the pot with the lid. Simmer the chickpeas for 30 minutes.

5. Turn the heat off. Stir in the spinach and parsley, and let the soup sit for 1 minute, until the spinach wilts. Squeeze half a lemon over the soup, stir and taste, adding more lemon juice to your liking.

6. Transfer the soup to serving bowls and top each bowl with a drizzle of olive oil and a bit of grated Pecorino Romano cheese. Serve with crusty bread.

Marinated White Bean and Tomato Salad

Ingredients:

• ½ cup extra-virgin olive oil

• 4 garlic cloves, thinly sliced

• Two 15.5-ounce cans white beans, such as butter beans or cannellini, drained and rinsed

• Zest of 1 lemon, finely grated

• 2 sprigs oregano, leaves removed (about 1 tablespoon fresh oregano leaves, or 2 tablespoons dried oregano)

• Kosher salt

• 2 pints cherry tomatoes or a couple large heirloom tomatoes, or a mix of shapes and sizes

Instructions:

1. In a small pot or skillet, place the oil and garlic and heat over medium-low until the garlic is just barely starting to turn golden brown and smells fragrant, about 5 minutes.

2. In a large bowl or resealable container, place the drained beans, pour the hot garlic oil over and toss to combine. Add the lemon zest and oregano and season to taste with salt. Let sit at least 1 hour at room temperature, or seal and transfer to the fridge overnight. About 1 hour before serving, remove from the fridge to bring up to room temperature so that the oil isn't cold and congealed.

3. At 30 minutes or 1 hour before serving, halve the cherry tomatoes (or cut the heirlooms into big bite-size pieces or wedges) and season liberally with salt. This helps intensify the tomato flavor (please don't skip this step).

4. Let them sit in a separate bowl from the beans until just before ready to serve, then lift the tomatoes out (leaving the juices behind) and toss them into the beans. Taste and adjust seasoning as needed.

5. If you want it to taste brighter, add a splash of sherry or red wine vinegar, and maybe add a few fresh oregano leaves. If you want a bit of spice, sprinkle in some crushed red pepper flakes. Transfer to a serving platter.

Baked Chicken and Ricotta Meatballs

Ingredients:

• 14 ounces (400g) broccolini, rough stems trimmed and thick pieces cut lengthwise

• 1 lemon, ends trimmed and thinly sliced

• 4 tablespoons extra-virgin olive oil, divided

• Kosher salt and freshly ground black pepper

• ½ teaspoon crushed red pepper flakes, or more if desired

• 1 large egg

• 2 garlic cloves, grated

• ¾ cup ricotta cheese, drained and lightly salted

- ½ cup parsley leaves and fine stems, roughly chopped

- ¾ cup panko breadcrumbs

- 1 pound ground chicken, preferably dark meat

- Juice of 1 lemon

- Grated Parmesan, for sprinkling (optional)

Instructions:

1. Preheat the oven to 425°F.

2. On a baking sheet, toss the broccoli and lemon slices with 3 tablespoons of the olive oil, salt, pepper and the red pepper flakes. Spread evenly on the baking sheet and set aside while you make the meatballs.

3. MAKE THE MEATBALLS: In a medium bowl, beat the egg, then add the garlic, ricotta, 1 teaspoon salt, parsley, pepper, the rest of the oil, breadcrumbs and meat, and use your hands to gently combine it (too much mushing will make them tough and dry). You should still see pieces of the meat through the seasonings.

4. Lightly wet your hands with water or oil and roll the meat into twenty loose (not tightly packed) rounds, slightly smaller than golf balls, using a gentle rolling motion between your hands (the water will keep them from sticking to your hands).

Set on large pieces of baking parchment on the counter to make for an easier clean up.

5. Nestle the meatballs on the baking sheet in between the broccoli and lemon. Bake until the meatballs are browned and cooked through and the broccoli is crispy, 15 to 20 minutes, shaking the baking sheet to move the meatballs and turning the tray around halfway to ensure even cooking.

6. Remove from the oven, squeeze the lemon juice on top and divide between plates. Finish with grated Parmesan, if using.

Mediterranean Couscous with Tuna and Pepperoncini

Ingredients:

COUSCOUS

• 1 cup chicken broth or water

• 1¼ cups couscous

• ¾ teaspoon kosher salt

ACCOMPANIMENTS

• Two 5-ounce cans oil packed tuna

• 1 pint cherry tomatoes, halved

• ½ cup sliced pepperoncini

- ⅓ cup chopped fresh parsley

- ¼ cup capers

- Extra-virgin olive oil, for serving

- Kosher salt and freshly ground black pepper

- 1 lemon, quartered

Instructions:

1. MAKE THE COUSCOUS: In a small pot, bring the broth or water to a boil over medium heat. Remove the pot from the heat, stir in the couscous and cover the pot. Let sit for 10 minutes.

2. MAKE THE ACCOMPANIMENTS: Meanwhile, in a medium bowl, toss together the tuna, tomatoes, pepperoncini, parsley and capers.

3. Fluff the couscous with a fork, season with salt and pepper, and drizzle with olive oil. Top the couscous with the tuna mixture and serve with lemon wedges.

One Skillet, Geek Sun-Dried Tomato Chicken and Farro

Ingredients:

* 2 tablespoons extra virgin olive oil

* 1-pound boneless, skinless chicken breasts, or small thighs

* 1/4 cup extra virgin olive oil

* 2 tablespoons balsamic vinegar

* 1 tablespoon chopped fresh dill

* 1 tablespoon chopped fresh oregano

* 1 tablespoon paprika

* 2 cloves garlic, minced or grated

* kosher salt and black pepper

* 1 cup uncooked farro or quinoa

* 2 1/2 cups low sodium chicken broth

* 2 cups baby spinach

* 1/2 cup oil packed sun-dried tomatoes

* 1/3 cup kalamata olives, pitted

* juice of 1 lemon

- 8 ounces feta cheese, cubed

- 1 tablespoon chopped fresh dill

- 3 tablespoons toasted pine nuts (optional)

Instructions:

1. Preheat the oven to 400 degrees F.

2. In a medium bowl, combine 2 tablespoons olive oil, the chicken, balsamic vinegar, dill, oregano, paprika, garlic, and a large pinch of both salt and pepper. Toss well to evenly coat the chicken.

3. Heat the remaining 2 tablespoons olive oil in a large dutch oven or cast-iron skillet, set over medium high heat. When the oil is shimmering, add the chicken and sear on both sides until golden, about 3-5 minutes per side. Remove the chicken from the skillet.

4. To the same skillet, add the farro. Cook 2-3 minutes. Add the chicken broth, spinach, sun-dried tomatoes, olives, and lemon juice. Bring to a boil over high heat and stir. Slide in the chicken and any juices left on the plate back into the skillet. Transfer to the oven and roast for 20 minutes or until the chicken is cooked through and the farro becomes soft.

5. Serve the chicken topped with feta, dill, and pine nuts.

Lemon Salmon with Garlic and Thyme

Ingredients:

• Four 5- to 6-ounce salmon fillets

• Extra virgin olive oil, as needed

• Kosher salt and freshly ground black pepper

• 1 whole lemon, zested and sliced into thin rounds

• ½ teaspoon dried thyme

• 4 to 5 five garlic cloves, peeled and lightly crushed

Instructions:

1. Preheat the oven to 400°F.

2. Place the salmon fillets in a baking dish, and drizzle lightly with olive oil. Season with salt and pepper, then sprinkle evenly with the lemon zest and thyme. Arrange the lemon slices on top of the fillets, and add the garlic cloves to the dish.

3. Transfer to the oven and bake until the salmon is cooked through and flakes with a fork, 18-20 minutes (adjust the baking time if your fillets are very thick or thin).

Ingredients:

- 1 tablespoon extra-virgin olive oil

- 1 red onion, thinly sliced

- 1 red bell pepper, thinly sliced

- 1 tablespoon fresh ginger, minced

- 3 garlic cloves, minced

- 1 small head cauliflower, cut into bite-size florets

- 2 teaspoons chili powder

- 1 teaspoon ground coriander

- 3 tablespoons red curry paste

- One 14-ounce can coconut milk

- 1 lime, halved

- One 28-ounce can chickpeas

- 1½ cups frozen peas

- Kosher salt and freshly ground black pepper

- Steamed rice, for serving (optional)

- ¼ cup chopped fresh cilantro

- 4 scallions, thinly sliced

Instructions:

1. In a large saucepan, heat the olive oil over medium heat. Add the onion and bell pepper, and sauté until nearly tender, about 5 minutes. Add the ginger and garlic, and sauté until fragrant, about 1 minute.

2. Add the cauliflower and toss well to combine. Stir in the chili powder, coriander and red curry paste, and cook until the mixture begins to caramelize, about 1 minute.

3. Stir in the coconut milk and bring the mixture to a simmer over medium-low heat. Cover the saucepan and continue to simmer until the cauliflower is tender, 8 to 10 minutes.

4. Remove the lid and squeeze lime juice into the curry, stirring well to combine. Add the chickpeas and peas, season with salt and pepper, and bring the mixture back to a simmer.

5. Serve with rice, if desired. Garnish each portion with 1 tablespoon cilantro and 1 tablespoon scallions.

Ingredients:

CRISPY CHICKPEAS

- One 28-ounce can chickpeas, drained

- 2 tablespoons extra-virgin olive oil

- Zest of 1 lemon

- 1 teaspoon smoked paprika

- Salt and freshly ground black pepper

DRESSING

- 4 anchovies

- 1 garlic clove, smashed

- ½ teaspoon salt

- 1 tablespoon Dijon mustard

- Juice of 1 lemon

- ½ cup extra-virgin olive oil

- ½ teaspoon freshly ground black pepper

KALE SALAD

- 1 large bunch Lacinato kale, shredded

- ⅓ cup Parmesan cheese

Instructions:

1. MAKE THE CRISPY CHICKPEAS: Preheat the oven to 400°F and line a baking sheet with parchment paper. In a large bowl, toss the chickpeas with the olive oil, lemon zest and paprika to combine. Season with salt and pepper.

2. Spread the chickpeas in an even layer on the prepared baking sheet and roast until very crisp, 40 to 45 minutes. Stir the chickpeas once or twice during cooking. Let cool to room temperature.

3. MAKE THE DRESSING: In a medium bowl, mash the anchovies, garlic and salt together to combine. Stir in the mustard and lemon juice; mix well.

1. 4, Add the olive oil gradually and whisk well to combine. Season with pepper.

4. ASSEMBLE THE SALAD: In a large bowl, toss the kale with the dressing. Top with the cooled chickpeas. Shave the Parmesan with a vegetable peeler to make large curls. Serve immediately.

Ingredients:

ALMOND SAUCE

- 2 tablespoons extra-virgin olive oil

- 3 shallots, minced

- 2 garlic cloves, minced

- 3 tablespoons all-purpose flour

- 2 cups plain, unsweetened almond milk

- 2 tablespoons Dijon mustard

- Salt and freshly ground black pepper

SWEET POTATO NOODLES

- 2 tablespoons extra-virgin olive oil

- 3 sweet potatoes, cut into noodles (made using a spiralizer)

- 4 cups roughly torn kale

- Salt and freshly ground black pepper

- ½ cup toasted, salted almonds, roughly chopped

Instructions:

1. MAKE THE ALMOND SAUCE: In a medium pot, heat the olive oil over medium heat. Add the shallots and garlic, and sauté until fragrant, about 1 minute.

2. Stir in the flour and cook, stirring constantly, for 1 minute. Add the almond milk, whisking constantly to prevent lumps from forming in the sauce. Whisk over medium heat until the mixture comes to a simmer. Simmer for 4 to 5 minutes.

3. Whisk in the Dijon mustard and season the sauce with salt and pepper. Cover and continue to warm the sauce over low heat while you prepare the noodles.

4. MAKE THE SWEET POTATO NOODLES: In a large sauté pan, heat the olive oil over medium heat. Add the sweet potato noodles and sauté, tossing occasionally, until they are nearly tender, 5 to 6 minutes.

5. Add the kale and toss until it wilts. Add the sauce and toss until the noodles are well coated.

6. Just before serving, add the almonds and toss to combine. Season with salt and pepper. Serve immediately.

Ingredients:

DRESSING

- ½ cup extra-virgin olive oil

- 1 tablespoon Dijon mustard

- 1 garlic clove, minced

- 1 teaspoon dried oregano

- 1 teaspoon salt

- ¾ teaspoon freshly ground black pepper

- ⅓ cup red wine vinegar

SALAD

- 1 head iceberg lettuce — washed, cored and quartered

- 1-pint cherry tomatoes, quartered

- ½ cucumber, thinly sliced

- ½ red onion, thinly sliced

- ½ cup crumbled feta cheese

- 1 cup kalamata olives

- 4 peperoncino peppers

Instructions:

1. MAKE THE DRESSING: In a medium bowl, whisk the olive oil with the mustard, garlic, oregano, salt and pepper. Gradually whisk in the red wine vinegar and mix well to combine.

2. MAKE THE SALAD: Place a quarter of iceberg lettuce on each plate and then sprinkle with an even amount of the tomatoes, cucumber and red onion. Drizzle each wedge with salad dressing to taste.

3. Garnish with 2 tablespoons feta, ¼ cup olives and a peperoncino pepper. Serve immediately.

Blistered Green Beans with Tomatoes, Pounded Walnuts and Raw Summer Squash

Ingredients:

- 1 cup walnuts, toasted

- ½ bunch parsley, roughly chopped

- Zest and juice of 1 lemon

- ¼ cup olive oil

• Kosher salt

• 1 tablespoon neutral oil, like canola

• 1-pound green beans, stems snapped off

• 1-pint cherry tomatoes, halved

• 1 medium summer squash, shaved into paper-thin planks or rounds

Instructions:

1. Place the walnuts in a ziplock plastic bag and bash with the bottom of a frying pan until the walnuts are broken into coarse pieces and have released some oil.

2. Combine the walnuts, parsley, lemon zest and juice, olive oil and a pinch of salt, and stir to combine.

3. Heat the neutral oil until smoking hot and add the green beans with a pinch of salt. Let the green beans blister, then toss to coat, flip and blister the other side.

4. Remove from the heat and toss with the tomatoes and summer squash. Top with the walnut mixture and serve.

Panzanella for One

Ingredients:

- 2 tablespoons extra-virgin olive oil

- 2½ teaspoons balsamic vinegar

- 1 garlic clove, minced

- ½ teaspoon dried oregano

- Kosher salt

- 1 cucumber, peeled and chopped

- 1 cup cubed stale bread (from a rustic country loaf or baguette)

- 1 cup chopped tomato

- 4 ounces feta cheese, crumbled

- ¼ cup chopped red onion

- 6 Kalamata olives, pitted and chopped

Instructions:

1. In a large bowl, combine the olive oil, vinegar, garlic, oregano and a pinch of salt. Whisk until emulsified. Add the cucumber, bread, tomato, feta, onion and olives.

2. Use your hands to toss the salad and evenly distribute the ingredients. Serve at room temperature.

Ingredients:

- 2 tablespoons extra-virgin olive oil

- 2 cups peeled pearl onions (frozen is fine)

- 3 celery stalks, chopped

- 3 garlic cloves, minced

- ½ cup white wine

- 1 tablespoon hot paprika

- Pinch cayenne pepper

- 2 tablespoons lemon zest

- Kosher salt

- Freshly ground black pepper

- One 28-ounce can crushed tomatoes

- 4 cups seafood or vegetable broth

- 2½ cups pasta

- 1½ pounds shrimp, peeled and deveined

- 3 cups roughly chopped kale

- Lemon zest, for garnish

- Chopped fresh parsley, for garnish

Instructions:

1. In a large pot, warm the olive oil over medium heat. Add the onions and celery and sauté until tender, 5 to 6 minutes. Add the garlic and continue to cook until fragrant, 1 minute more.

2. Add the wine and bring to a simmer. Cook until the liquid is reduced by about half, 6 to 7 minutes. Season with paprika, cayenne pepper, lemon zest, salt and pepper. Simmer until fragrant, 1 to 2 minutes more.

3. Add the tomatoes and broth and return to a simmer. Stir in the pasta and cook until it just starts to become tender, 5 minutes. Reduce the heat to low, add the shrimp and kale and continue to simmer over very low heat until the pasta is tender, the shrimp are cooked through and the kale is wilted, 4 to 5 minutes.

4. To serve, ladle the stew into bowls and garnish generously with lemon zest and parsley. Serve with crusty bread.

Ingredients:

LEMON-HERB SAUCE

- 1 cup parsley leaves

- ½ cup cilantro leaves

- ½ cup mint leaves

- ½ cup roughly chopped green onion

- 1 garlic clove, smashed

- Juice of 1 lemon

- ⅓ cup olive oil

CAULIFLOWER STEAKS

- 1 large head cauliflower

- 4 tablespoons extra-virgin olive oil, divided

- 4 teaspoons smoked paprika

- Salt and freshly ground black pepper, to taste

Instructions:

1. MAKE THE HERB SAUCE: In a blender or food processor, pulse the parsley, cilantro, mint, green onion, garlic, lemon juice and olive oil until completely smooth. Set aside.

2. MAKE THE CAULIFLOWER STEAKS: With a sharp knife, cut the cauliflower into 1-inch-thick slices. (You should get about 8 slices.) Rub both sides of each piece of cauliflower with about 1 teaspoon olive oil. Sprinkle both sides of each piece with ½ teaspoon smoked paprika, salt and pepper.

3. Heat the remaining 1 tablespoon olive oil in a large cast-iron skillet over medium-high heat. Working in batches, sear the cauliflower steaks until they are golden brown, 3 to 4 minutes per side. The cauliflower should be easily pierced with a fork but not so tender that it falls apart.

4. To serve, place 2 cauliflower steaks on each plate and top with a generous drizzle of the lemon-herb sauce. Serve immediately.

Kamut and Sour Cherry Meze

Ingredients:

• 1 cup kamut

• ½ cup chopped dried sour cherries

- ⅓ cup finely chopped toasted walnuts

- ⅓ cup finely chopped fresh parsley

- ¼ cup finely chopped red onion

- ¼ cup finely chopped fresh dill, plus more sprigs for serving

- 2 tablespoons extra-virgin olive oil

- 1 tablespoon lemon juice

- 1 garlic clove, grated

- 1 teaspoon kosher teaspoon salt

- ¼ teaspoon freshly ground black pepper

- ¼ cup feta cheese

Instructions:

1. Bring 3 cups of salted water to a boil, add the Kamut, cover and reduce the heat to a simmer. Cook until tender, about 50 to 60 minutes.

2. Toss the Kamut with the cherries, walnuts, parsley, red onion and dill.

3. In a medium bowl, whisk together the olive oil, lemon juice, garlic, salt and pepper. Drizzle the dressing over the Kamut and garnish with the feta and dill sprigs.

Ingredients:

• 1 bunch broccoli rabe, tips of stems trimmed off

• 1 to 2 tablespoons extra-virgin olive oil, plus more for drizzling

• 2 garlic cloves, sliced

• ¼ teaspoon red-pepper flakes

• 4 ounces burrata or fresh mozzarella

• ½ tablespoon fresh lemon juice

• 2 tablespoons crushed, toasted pistachios

• Flaky sea salt, for serving

Instructions:

1. Bring a large pot of salted water to a boil. Boil the broccoli rabe for 3 minutes, then drain.

2. In a large, deep skillet over medium heat, heat enough olive oil to nicely coat the bottom of the pan, 1 to 2 tablespoons. Stir in the garlic and cook for 30 seconds, then stir in the red-pepper flakes.

3. Add the broccoli rabe and sauté, shaking the pan and gently tossing so that it cooks evenly, until tender (especially the stems), 3 to 5 minutes.

4. Remove the broccoli rabe from the pan and drain off any excess liquid. Arrange the broccoli on a plate or platter. Tear the burrata and scatter the pieces among the broccoli rabe. Sprinkle with lemon juice, pistachios and salt. Drizzle with olive oil, if desired, and serve.

Honey-Lime Chicken and Veggies in Foil

Ingredients:

- 3 tablespoons unsalted butter, melted

- 2 tablespoons extra-virgin olive oil

- 2 garlic cloves, minced

- 1 tablespoon minced ginger

- 2 tablespoons honey

- Zest of 1 lime

- Four 6-ounce chicken breasts

- 1 teaspoon cumin

- ½ teaspoon smoked paprika

- 1 bunch asparagus

- Kosher salt and freshly ground black pepper

- 2 ears corn, halved

- 2 tablespoons chopped fresh cilantro

- ¼ cup thinly sliced green onion

Instructions:

1. In a small bowl, stir together the butter, olive oil, garlic, ginger, honey and lime zest.

2. Using 12-inch sheets of foil, build four packets. Place a chicken breast in the center of each. Season it with cumin and paprika. Divide the asparagus among the packets. Brush the chicken and asparagus with the honey-ginger sauce and season with salt and pepper. Fold the foil over the food inside and crimp several times to seal.

3. Preheat a grill or grill pan over medium-high heat. Grill the packets until the chicken is cooked through, 10 to 12 minutes.

4. About 5 minutes before the chicken is finished, add the corn to the grill and cook until it's browned on all sides, about 5 minutes.

5. Garnish the chicken with cilantro and green onion before serving.

Ingredients:

GARLIC OIL

- ⅓ cup extra-virgin olive oil

- 3 garlic cloves, thinly sliced

SKEWERS

- 3 cups sourdough bread, cubed

- 3 cups cubed halloumi

- 4 cups cherry tomatoes

- Salt and freshly ground black pepper

- ¾ cup basil leaves

- Balsamic vinegar, as needed

Instructions:

1. MAKE THE GARLIC OIL: Combine the oil and garlic and heat gently over medium-low heat for 2 to 3 minutes. Let cool completely and then remove the garlic from the oil.

2. MAKE THE SKEWERS: Arrange 2 or 3 pieces of bread, 3 or 4 pieces of cheese and 3 or 4 tomatoes on each skewer. Repeat until all the skewers are assembled.

3. Brush the skewers with the garlic oil on both sides and season with salt and pepper. Working in batches, cook on a preheated grill or grill pan until nicely charred on both sides, 2 to 3 minutes per side.

4. Add a few basil leaves to the end of each skewer and then roughly chop the remaining basil and garnish the skewers with the chopped basil.

5. Serve the skewers immediately, drizzled with balsamic vinegar.

Guacamole Quinoa Salad

Ingredients:

• 1 cup quinoa, rinsed

• 2 avocados, halved and pitted

• ½ small white or red onion, finely diced

• ½ cup loosely packed chopped fresh cilantro

• 2 tablespoons freshly squeezed lime juice

- ½ teaspoon kosher salt

- One 15-ounce can black beans, drained and rinsed

- 1 cup cherry tomatoes, quartered

- Extra-virgin olive oil, for drizzling

- Romaine lettuce, minced garlic, hot sauce, red-pepper flakes and lime wedges, for serving

Instructions:

1. Cook the quinoa according to package instructions. Allow it to cool to room temperature.

2. Score the avocado flesh (still in the skin) with a paring knife, then scoop the flesh into a large bowl. Coarsely mash about half of the avocado with a fork, leaving plenty of chunks intact. Mix in the onion, cilantro, lime juice and salt.

3. Gently fold in the black beans, tomatoes and quinoa. Taste and adjust the seasonings if desired and drizzle with olive oil.

4. Serve on a bed of romaine lettuce topped with garlic, hot sauce and red-pepper flakes alongside lime wedges.

CHAPTER THREE

DESSERT RECIPES

Berry and Yogurt Parfait

Ingredients:

• 1 cup Greek yogurt (unsweetened)

• 1 cup mixed berries (strawberries, blueberries, raspberries)

• 2 tablespoons honey or maple syrup (optional)

• 1/4 cup granola (optional)

• Fresh mint leaves for garnish

Instructions:

1. Wash and dry the mixed berries. Slice strawberries if desired.

2. In serving glasses or bowls, layer Greek yogurt, mixed berries, and honey or maple syrup if using. Repeat the layers as desired.

3. Optionally, add a layer of granola between the yogurt and berries for texture.

4. Top with a few fresh mint leaves for garnish before serving.

Dark Chocolate-Dipped Strawberries

Ingredients:

• Fresh strawberries

• Dark chocolate (70% cocoa or higher)

• Chopped nuts (optional)

Instructions:

1. Wash and thoroughly dry the strawberries. Leave the stems intact.

2. Break the dark chocolate into pieces and melt it in a heatproof bowl over a pot of simmering water, stirring occasionally until smooth.

3. Dip each strawberry into the melted chocolate, covering about two-thirds of the berry. Allow excess chocolate to drip back into the bowl.

4. If desired, roll the chocolate-dipped strawberries in chopped nuts before the chocolate sets.

5. Place the dipped strawberries on a parchment-lined tray and refrigerate until the chocolate hardens.

Banana Oatmeal Cookies

Ingredients:

• 2 ripe bananas

• 1 cup rolled oats

• 1/4 cup chopped nuts or seeds (such as walnuts or sunflower seeds)

• 1/4 cup raisins or dried cranberries (optional)

• 1 teaspoon cinnamon

• 1/2 teaspoon vanilla extract (optional)

Instructions:

1. Preheat the oven to 350°F (175°C). Line a baking sheet with parchment paper.

2. In a bowl, mash the ripe bananas until smooth.

3. Add rolled oats, chopped nuts or seeds, raisins or dried cranberries if using, cinnamon, and vanilla extract to the mashed bananas. Mix until well combined.

4. Scoop spoonfuls of the mixture and place them on the prepared baking sheet, flattening each slightly with the back of the spoon.

5. Bake in the preheated oven for about 12-15 minutes or until the cookies are lightly golden.

6. Allow the cookies to cool on the baking sheet for a few minutes before transferring them to a wire rack to cool completely.

Chia Seed Pudding

Ingredients:

• 1/4 cup chia seeds

• 1 cup unsweetened almond milk or any preferred milk

• 1 tablespoon honey or maple syrup (optional)

• Fresh fruit for topping (such as sliced strawberries, blueberries, or mango)

Instructions:

1. In a bowl or jar, mix chia seeds and almond milk. Add honey or maple syrup if desired. Stir well.

2. Cover the bowl or jar and refrigerate for at least 2 hours, or overnight, to allow the chia seeds to absorb the liquid and form a pudding-like consistency.

3. Before serving, stir the chia pudding mixture to break up any clumps.

4. Top with fresh fruit before serving.

Apple Cinnamon Baked Oatmeal Cups

Ingredients:

• 2 cups rolled oats

• 2 ripe bananas (mashed)

• 2 apples (peeled and diced)

• 1 teaspoon cinnamon

• 1/4 cup chopped nuts (optional)

• 1 tablespoon honey or maple syrup (optional)

• 1 1/2 cups unsweetened almond milk or any preferred milk

Instructions:

1. Preheat the oven to 350°F (175°C). Grease a muffin tin or line it with paper liners.

2. In a bowl, combine rolled oats, mashed bananas, diced apples, cinnamon, chopped nuts if using, honey or maple syrup

if desired, and unsweetened almond milk. Mix until well combined.

3. Spoon the oatmeal mixture into the prepared muffin tin, filling each cup almost to the top.

4. Bake in the preheated oven for about 25-30 minutes or until the oatmeal cups are set and lightly golden on top.

5. Allow the oatmeal cups to cool slightly before removing them from the muffin tin. Serve warm or at room temperature.

Mixed Berry Frozen Yogurt Bark

Ingredients:

• 2 cups Greek yogurt (unsweetened)

• 1 tablespoon honey or maple syrup

• 1 cup mixed berries (strawberries, blueberries, raspberries)

• 2 tablespoons unsweetened shredded coconut (optional)

• Parchment paper

Instructions:

1. In a bowl, combine Greek yogurt with honey or maple syrup.

2. Wash and dry the mixed berries. Slice larger berries if desired.

3. Line a baking sheet with parchment paper. Spread the sweetened yogurt evenly on the parchment paper, creating a rectangular shape.

4. Sprinkle the mixed berries and shredded coconut evenly over the yogurt.

5. Place the baking sheet in the freezer for at least 3-4 hours or until the yogurt bark is frozen solid.

6. Once frozen, break the bark into pieces and serve immediately as a refreshing dessert.

Almond Butter Banana Bites

Ingredients:

• Bananas (firm, not overly ripe)

• Almond butter (or any nut or seed butter)

• Dark chocolate chips (70% cocoa or higher)

Instructions:

1. Peel and slice the bananas into rounds, about 1/2-inch thick.

2. Spread a small amount of almond butter on one side of each banana round.

3. Create mini "sandwiches" by placing another banana round on top, making a banana-almond butter sandwich.

4. Melt dark chocolate chips in a microwave-safe bowl in short intervals, stirring until smooth.

5. Dip half of each banana-almond butter sandwich into the melted chocolate.

6. Place the dipped banana bites on a parchment-lined tray and freeze until the chocolate hardens.

7. Once the chocolate is firm, serve the almond butter banana bites.

Cinnamon Baked Apples

Ingredients:

- 4 apples (any baking variety)

- 1/4 cup chopped nuts (such as walnuts or pecans)

- 2 tablespoons honey or maple syrup

- 1 teaspoon cinnamon

- 1 tablespoon unsalted butter (or coconut oil)

- Lemon juice (from half a lemon)

- Optional: Greek yogurt or whipped cream for serving

Instructions:

1. Preheat the oven to 375°F (190°C).

2. Core the apples, leaving the bottom intact to form a cavity for the filling.

3. In a bowl, mix chopped nuts, honey or maple syrup, cinnamon, unsalted butter (or coconut oil), and a splash of lemon juice.

4. Stuff the apple cavities with the nut mixture.

5. Place the stuffed apples in a baking dish and bake for about 25-30 minutes or until apples are tender.

6. Serve the cinnamon baked apples warm, optionally topped with a dollop of Greek yogurt or whipped cream.

Mango Coconut Chia Popsicles

Ingredients:

- 1 ripe mango (peeled and diced)

- 1 can (13.5 oz) coconut milk (full-fat)

• 2 tablespoons honey or maple syrup

• 1/4 cup chia seeds

Instructions:

1. In a blender, blend diced mango, coconut milk, and honey or maple syrup until smooth.

2. Pour the mango-coconut mixture into a bowl and stir in chia seeds. Mix well.

3. Pour the mixture into popsicle molds.

4. Place the molds in the freezer for at least 4-6 hours or until the popsicles are frozen solid.

5. Run the molds under warm water for a few seconds to release the popsicles. Serve and enjoy.

Baked Peaches with Honey and Cinnamon

Ingredients:

• 4 ripe peaches (halved and pitted)

• 2 tablespoons honey

• 1 teaspoon cinnamon

• Optional: Greek yogurt or vanilla ice cream for serving

Instructions:

1. Preheat the oven to 375°F (190°C).

2. Cut the peaches in half and remove the pits. Place the peach halves, cut side up, on a baking sheet lined with parchment paper.

3. Drizzle honey over the peach halves and sprinkle them with cinnamon.

4. Bake in the preheated oven for about 20-25 minutes or until the peaches are tender and caramelized.

5. Serve the baked peaches warm, optionally topped with a dollop of Greek yogurt or a scoop of vanilla ice cream.

Blueberry Chia Seed Pudding Cups

Ingredients:

• 1/4 cup chia seeds

• 1 cup unsweetened almond milk (or any preferred milk)

• 1 tablespoon honey or maple syrup

• 1 cup fresh blueberries

• 1 tablespoon unsweetened shredded coconut (optional)

• Fresh mint leaves for garnish

Instructions:

1. In a bowl or jar, combine chia seeds, almond milk, and honey or maple syrup. Stir well.

2. Let it sit in the refrigerator for at least 2 hours or until the mixture thickens to a pudding-like consistency.

3. Once the chia seed pudding is ready, layer it with fresh blueberries in serving cups or jars.

4. Optionally, sprinkle unsweetened shredded coconut on top.

5. Garnish with fresh mint leaves before serving.

Baked Cinnamon Apple Chips

Ingredients:

• 2 apples (any baking variety)

• 1 teaspoon cinnamon

• Optional: 1 tablespoon honey

Instructions:

1. Preheat the oven to 200°F (95°C). Line baking sheets with parchment paper.

2. Core the apples and thinly slice them crosswise using a sharp knife or mandoline slicer.

3. In a bowl, toss the apple slices with cinnamon. Add honey for extra sweetness if desired.

4. Place the apple slices on the prepared baking sheets in a single layer, making sure they don't overlap.

5. Bake for about 2-3 hours, flipping the slices halfway through, until the apples are dried and crispy.

6. Allow the apple chips to cool completely before serving as a crispy and naturally sweet snack.

Mango Sorbet

Ingredients:

• 3 ripe mangoes (peeled and diced)

• 1-2 tablespoons honey or maple syrup (optional)

• Juice of 1 lime or lemon

Instructions:

1. Place the diced mangoes in a single layer on a baking sheet lined with parchment paper.

2. Freeze for at least 2 hours or until solid.

3. In a food processor or blender, blend the frozen mango chunks until smooth.

4. Add honey or maple syrup and lime or lemon juice if desired for added sweetness and tang.

5. Transfer the mango puree to a container and freeze for an additional 30-60 minutes for a firmer sorbet, or serve immediately for a softer consistency.

Walnut Date Energy Balls

Ingredients:

• 1 cup dates (pitted)

• 1 cup walnuts

• 2 tablespoons unsweetened cocoa powder

• 1 tablespoon coconut oil

• Shredded coconut for rolling (optional)

Instructions:

1. In a food processor, combine pitted dates, walnuts, cocoa powder, and coconut oil.

2. Pulse until the mixture forms a sticky dough-like consistency.

3. Take small portions of the mixture and roll them into bite-sized balls using your hands.

4. Roll the energy balls in shredded coconut for an extra layer of flavor (optional).

5. Place the energy balls in the refrigerator for about 30 minutes to set. Enjoy these nutritious and naturally sweet energy balls as a snack or dessert.

Raspberry Greek Yogurt Popsicles

Ingredients:

• 1 cup Greek yogurt (unsweetened)

• 1 cup fresh raspberries

• 2 tablespoons honey or maple syrup

• Popsicle molds and sticks

Instructions:

1. In a blender, combine Greek yogurt, fresh raspberries, and honey or maple syrup. Blend until smooth.

2. Pour the mixture into popsicle molds.

3. Insert popsicle sticks into the molds and freeze for at least 4 hours or until the popsicles are frozen solid.

4. Run the molds under warm water for a few seconds to release the popsicles. Serve and enjoy these refreshing treats.

Lemon Blueberry Chia Seed Muffins

Ingredients:

- 1 1/2 cups almond flour

- 1/4 cup chia seeds

- 1 teaspoon baking powder

- 1/4 teaspoon salt

- 2 tablespoons coconut oil (melted)

- 1/4 cup honey or maple syrup

- 2 large eggs

- Zest of 1 lemon

- 1/4 cup fresh blueberries

Instructions:

1. Preheat the oven to 350°F (175°C). Line a muffin tin with paper liners.

2. In a bowl, combine almond flour, chia seeds, baking powder, and salt.

3. In another bowl, whisk together melted coconut oil, honey or maple syrup, eggs, and lemon zest.

4. Gradually mix the wet ingredients into the dry ingredients until well combined. Gently fold in fresh blueberries.

5. Spoon the batter into the prepared muffin tin, filling each cup about 2/3 full.

6. Bake for 20-25 minutes or until a toothpick inserted into the center of a muffin comes out clean.

7. Allow the muffins to cool in the tin for a few minutes before transferring them to a wire rack to cool completely.

Coconut Rice Pudding with Mango

Ingredients:

• 1 cup cooked brown rice

• 1 can (13.5 oz) coconut milk (full-fat)

• 2 tablespoons honey or maple syrup

• 1 teaspoon vanilla extract

• 1 ripe mango (peeled and diced)

• Unsweetened shredded coconut for garnish

Instructions:

1. In a saucepan, combine cooked brown rice, coconut milk, honey or maple syrup, and vanilla extract.

2. Cook over medium-low heat, stirring occasionally, until the mixture thickens (about 20-25 minutes).

3. Remove the rice pudding from heat and let it cool to room temperature. Then refrigerate until chilled.

4. Spoon the coconut rice pudding into serving bowls and top with diced mango.

5. Garnish with unsweetened shredded coconut before serving.

Chocolate Avocado Mousse

Ingredients:

• 2 ripe avocados

• 1/4 cup unsweetened cocoa powder

• 1/4 cup honey or maple syrup

• 1 teaspoon vanilla extract

• Pinch of salt

• Fresh berries for topping (optional)

Instructions:

1. Scoop the flesh of ripe avocados into a blender or food processor.

2. Add cocoa powder, honey or maple syrup, vanilla extract, and a pinch of salt. Blend until smooth and creamy.

3. Transfer the chocolate avocado mousse to serving cups or bowls and refrigerate for at least 30 minutes to chill.

4. Top with fresh berries if desired before serving.

Almond Flour Banana Bread

Ingredients:

• 2 cups almond flour

• 1 teaspoon baking powder

• 1/2 teaspoon baking soda

• Pinch of salt

• 3 ripe bananas (mashed)

• 1/4 cup honey or maple syrup

- 1/4 cup coconut oil (melted)

- 2 large eggs

- 1 teaspoon vanilla extract

- Optional: Chopped nuts for topping

Instructions:

1. Preheat the oven to 350°F (175°C). Grease a loaf pan.

2. In a bowl, combine almond flour, baking powder, baking soda, and a pinch of salt.

3. In another bowl, mix mashed bananas, honey or maple syrup, melted coconut oil, eggs, and vanilla extract.

4. Gradually add the wet ingredients to the dry ingredients and stir until just combined.

5. Pour the batter into the prepared loaf pan. Optionally, sprinkle chopped nuts on top.

6. Bake for 45-55 minutes or until a toothpick inserted into the center comes out clean.

7. Allow the banana bread to cool in the pan for 10 minutes before transferring it to a wire rack to cool completely. Slice and serve.

Ingredients:

- 2 ripe bananas (peeled, sliced, and frozen)

- 1 cup fresh strawberries (hulled and frozen)

- 1-2 tablespoons honey or maple syrup (optional)

- Fresh strawberries for garnish (optional)

Instructions:

1. Place frozen banana slices and frozen strawberries in a blender or food processor.

2. Blend until smooth and creamy, scraping down the sides as needed.

3. Add honey or maple syrup if a sweeter taste is desired, then blend again to combine.

4. Scoop the strawberry banana nice cream into bowls. Garnish with fresh strawberry slices if desired and enjoy immediately.

Apple Cinnamon Quinoa Breakfast Bars

Ingredients:

• 1 cup cooked quinoa

• 2 cups rolled oats

• 2 apples (peeled, cored, and diced)

• 1/4 cup honey or maple syrup

• 1 teaspoon cinnamon

• 1/4 cup chopped nuts (such as walnuts or almonds)

• 1/4 cup raisins or dried cranberries

• 2 eggs

• 1 teaspoon vanilla extract

Instructions:

1. Preheat the oven to 350°F (175°C). Grease a baking dish or line it with parchment paper.

2. In a large bowl, combine cooked quinoa, rolled oats, diced apples, honey or maple syrup, cinnamon, chopped nuts, and raisins or dried cranberries.

3. In a separate bowl, beat the eggs and vanilla extract together. Pour this mixture into the dry ingredients and mix until well combined.

4. Transfer the mixture into the prepared baking dish, spreading it evenly.

5. Bake for 25-30 minutes or until golden brown and set.

6. Allow the bars to cool in the dish before slicing into squares or bars.

Oatmeal Raisin Cookies

Ingredients:

- 1 1/2 cups rolled oats

- 1 cup almond flour

- 1/2 teaspoon baking soda

- 1/2 teaspoon ground cinnamon

- Pinch of salt

- 1/4 cup coconut oil (melted)

- 1/4 cup honey or maple syrup

- 1 egg

- 1 teaspoon vanilla extract

- 1/2 cup raisins

Instructions:

1. Preheat the oven to 350°F (175°C). Line a baking sheet with parchment paper.

2. In a bowl, combine rolled oats, almond flour, baking soda, ground cinnamon, and a pinch of salt.

3. In another bowl, whisk together melted coconut oil, honey or maple syrup, egg, and vanilla extract.

4. Gradually mix the wet ingredients into the dry ingredients until well combined. Fold in the raisins.

5. Drop spoonfuls of dough onto the prepared baking sheet, flattening each slightly with the back of the spoon.

6. Bake for 12-15 minutes or until the cookies are golden brown.

7. Allow the cookies to cool on the baking sheet for a few minutes before transferring them to a wire rack to cool completely.

Peach and Berry Fruit Salad

Ingredients:

• 2 peaches (sliced)

• 1 cup fresh berries (such as strawberries, blueberries, raspberries)

• 1 tablespoon honey

• Juice of 1/2 lemon

• Fresh mint leaves for garnish

Instructions:

1. Slice the peaches and wash the berries.

2. In a bowl, combine sliced peaches and fresh berries.

3. Drizzle honey and squeeze lemon juice over the fruit. Gently toss until the fruit is coated.

4. Refrigerate the fruit salad for about 30 minutes before serving. Garnish with fresh mint leaves before serving.

Carrot Cake Energy Bites

Ingredients:

• 1 cup rolled oats

• 1/2 cup shredded carrots

• 1/4 cup almond butter

• 1/4 cup honey or maple syrup

• 1/4 cup chopped nuts (such as walnuts or pecans)

• 1 teaspoon cinnamon

• 1/2 teaspoon vanilla extract

• Shredded coconut for coating (optional)

Instructions:

1. In a bowl, combine rolled oats, shredded carrots, almond butter, honey or maple syrup, chopped nuts, cinnamon, and vanilla extract.

2. Use your hands to roll the mixture into bite-sized balls.

3. Roll the energy bites in shredded coconut for an additional layer (optional).

4. Place the carrot cake energy bites in the refrigerator for at least 30 minutes to firm up.

5. Enjoy these nutritious energy bites as a snack or dessert.

Almond Butter Stuffed Dates

Ingredients:

• Medjool dates (pitted)

• Almond butter (or any nut or seed butter)

• Optional: Chopped nuts, shredded coconut, or dark chocolate chips for topping

Instructions:

1. Make a small slit lengthwise in each date and remove the pit.

2. Spoon a small amount of almond butter (or preferred nut/seed butter) into each date.

3. Optionally, top each stuffed date with chopped nuts, shredded coconut, or a dark chocolate chip.

4. Arrange the almond butter stuffed dates on a plate and serve as a naturally sweet treat.

Frozen Banana Pops

Ingredients:

• Ripe bananas

• Wooden popsicle sticks

• Toppings: Melted dark chocolate, chopped nuts, shredded coconut, or dried fruits

Instructions:

1. Peel bananas and cut them in half crosswise.

2. Insert a wooden popsicle stick into the cut end of each banana half.

3. Place the banana pops on a parchment-lined tray and freeze for at least 1 hour or until solid.

4. Dip each frozen banana pop into melted dark chocolate or preferred coating.

5. Optionally, roll the coated banana pops in chopped nuts, shredded coconut, or dried fruits before the coating sets.

6. Place the coated banana pops back in the freezer for a few minutes to set the coating completely.

7. Serve these frozen banana pops as a refreshing and healthy dessert.

Baked Pear with Cinnamon and Honey

Ingredients:

• Pears (halved and cored)

• 1 tablespoon honey

• Ground cinnamon

• Optional: Chopped nuts or Greek yogurt for serving

Instructions:

1. Preheat the oven to 375°F (190°C).

2. Place the halved and cored pears on a baking sheet or in a baking dish, cut side up.

3. Drizzle honey over the pears and sprinkle them with ground cinnamon.

4. Bake for 20-25 minutes or until the pears are tender and caramelized.

5. Serve the baked pears warm, optionally topped with chopped nuts or a dollop of Greek yogurt.

Blueberry Coconut Chia Popsicles

Ingredients:

• 1 cup fresh blueberries

• 1 can (13.5 oz) coconut milk (full-fat)

• 2 tablespoons honey or maple syrup

• 1/4 cup chia seeds

Instructions:

1. In a blender, blend fresh blueberries and coconut milk until smooth.

2. Pour the blueberry-coconut mixture into a bowl and stir in chia seeds. Mix well.

3. Pour the mixture into popsicle molds.

4. Insert popsicle sticks into the molds and freeze for at least 4 hours or until the popsicles are frozen solid.

5. Run the molds under warm water for a few seconds to release the popsicles. Serve and enjoy.

Raspberry Yogurt Parfait Cups

Ingredients:

• Greek yogurt (unsweetened)

• Fresh raspberries

• Granola

• Optional: Drizzle of honey or maple syrup

Instructions:

1. In serving cups or jars, layer Greek yogurt, fresh raspberries, and granola.

2. Optionally, drizzle a bit of honey or maple syrup between the layers for sweetness.

3. Repeat the layers as desired, ending with a layer of granola on top.

4. Serve these raspberry yogurt parfaits as a delightful and nutritious dessert.

Ingredients:

Chocolate Peanut Butter Swirl

- ½ cup canned pumpkin

- 1/2 cup creamy all-natural peanut butter

- 3 tablespoons maple syrup

- 1 tsp chocolate extract

- 1.5 Tbs Organic Dutch Process Cocoa

Pumpkin Pie Bar

- 1/2 cup quick oats

- 2 tsp pumpkin pie spice or 1 tsp cinnamon + 1/4 tsp nutmeg

- 1 1/2 tsp baking powder

- 1/4 teaspoon Kosher salt

- 1 1/2 cups white beans, cannellini or another soft white bean (1 15-oz can, drained and rinsed)

- 1/2 cup canned pumpkin

- 1/3 cup pure maple syrup

• 1.5 tsp Pumpkin Spice Extract

Instructions

1. Preheat oven to 350 F. Lightly grease an 8×8 baking pan.

2. In a small bowl, combine all the swirl ingredients, mix until well combined. Set aside.

3. In the bowl of a Cuisinart mixer, blend the oats, pumpkin pie spice, baking powder and salt until just combined - just a few pulses so they're evenly distributed.

4. Add bean, pumpkin, maple syrup and extract. Blend until very smooth.

5. Empty the Cuisinart mixer bowl into the prepared glass baking dish. Use a spatula to evenly distribute and smooth the batter.

6. Starting in one corner, use a small spoon to scoop about 1 Tbs of chocolate pumpkin swirl batter onto the top. You'll dollop 4 scoops across and 4 scoops down making a total of 16 dollops.

7. Using the tip of a knife, swirl the two batters together. They will be on the thick side, so it won't be a perfect swirl, but any swirly pattern looks scrumptious to me!

8. Bake for 35 minutes. You want the top dry and the edges to start to pull away from the sides. It shouldn't be jiggly when

shaken, but it will still be slightly soft inside - like pumpkin pie - these pumpkin pie bars will firm up as they cool.

9. Let cool at least 1 hour before trying to cut. They will have a firm edge, soft pumpkin pie middle and chunks of chocolate peanut butter on the top.

10. Store in fridge or freezer.

Green Tea with Lemon and Honey

Ingredients:

- 1 green tea bag

- 1 cup hot water

- 1 teaspoon honey (optional)

- Fresh lemon slices

Instructions:

1. Place a green tea bag in a cup and pour hot water over it.

2. Let the tea steep for 2-3 minutes, or as per package instructions.

3. Add honey if desired and stir until dissolved. Squeeze a fresh lemon slice into the tea and stir gently.

4. Remove the tea bag and serve the green tea hot.

Berry and Spinach Smoothie

Ingredients:

• 1 cup fresh spinach

• 1/2 cup mixed berries (such as strawberries, blueberries, raspberries)

• 1/2 banana

• 1/2 cup Greek yogurt (unsweetened)

• 1/2 cup almond milk (unsweetened)

• 1 tablespoon chia seeds (optional)

• Ice cubes (optional)

Instructions:

1. In a blender, combine fresh spinach, mixed berries, banana, Greek yogurt, almond milk, and chia seeds.

2. Blend until the mixture reaches a smooth consistency.

3. If desired, add ice cubes and blend until incorporated.

4. Pour the smoothie into a glass and enjoy this nutrient-rich beverage.

Turmeric Golden Milk

Ingredients:

• 1 cup unsweetened almond milk (or any preferred milk)

• 1/2 teaspoon ground turmeric

• 1/4 teaspoon ground cinnamon

• 1/4 teaspoon ground ginger

• Pinch of ground black pepper

• 1 teaspoon honey or maple syrup (optional)

• 1/2 teaspoon coconut oil (optional)

Instructions:

1. In a small saucepan, heat almond milk over medium-low heat. Stir in ground turmeric, cinnamon, ginger, and black pepper.

2. Add honey or maple syrup for sweetness, if desired.

3. Optionally, add coconut oil and stir until melted.

4. Simmer the mixture for a few minutes while stirring occasionally. Strain through a fine-mesh sieve if desired.

5. Pour the turmeric golden milk into a cup and savor this comforting and anti-inflammatory beverage.

Citrus Infused Water

Ingredients:

- 1 lemon (sliced)

- 1 lime (sliced)

- 1 orange (sliced)

- Fresh mint leaves

- Ice cubes

- Water

Instructions:

1. Slice the lemon, lime, and orange into thin rounds.

2. In a pitcher, place the citrus slices and a few fresh mint leaves. Add ice cubes and fill the pitcher with water.

3. Let the mixture sit in the refrigerator for at least an hour to infuse flavors.

4. Pour the citrus-infused water into glasses, ensuring each serving has citrus slices and mint leaves.

Herbal Iced Tea with Berries

Ingredients:

• Herbal tea bags (such as chamomile, peppermint, or hibiscus)

• Mixed berries (strawberries, raspberries, blueberries)

• Fresh mint leaves

• Honey or maple syrup (optional)

• Ice cubes

Instructions:

1. Brew herbal tea bags according to package instructions and let it cool to room temperature.

2. In a pitcher, muddle a handful of mixed berries and a few fresh mint leaves to release flavors.

3. Pour the cooled herbal tea into the pitcher with the muddled berries and mint.

4. Add honey or maple syrup for sweetness if desired. Stir well and refrigerate to chill.

5. Fill glasses with ice cubes and pour the herbal berry tea over the ice.

6. Garnish with additional fresh berries or mint leaves before serving.

Kale Pineapple Smoothie

Ingredients:

• 1 cup kale leaves (stems removed)

• 1 cup fresh pineapple chunks

• 1/2 banana

• 1/2 cup unsweetened almond milk

• 1 tablespoon Greek yogurt (unsweetened)

• Optional: 1 tablespoon chia seeds or flaxseeds

Instructions:

1. In a blender, combine kale leaves, pineapple chunks, banana, almond milk, Greek yogurt, and chia seeds or flaxseeds.

2. Blend until the mixture becomes smooth and creamy.

3. Pour the kale pineapple smoothie into a glass and enjoy this nutrient-packed beverage.

Cucumber Mint Infused Water

Ingredients:

• 1 cucumber (sliced)

• Fresh mint leaves

• Ice cubes

• Water

Instructions:

1. Slice the cucumber into thin rounds and tear a few fresh mint leaves.

2. In a pitcher, place the cucumber slices and torn mint leaves. Add ice cubes and fill the pitcher with water.

3. Allow the pitcher to sit in the refrigerator for a few hours to infuse flavors.

4. Pour the cucumber mint infused water into glasses, ensuring each serving has cucumber slices and mint leaves.

Ginger Turmeric Lemonade

Ingredients:

• 4 cups water

• 1 tablespoon fresh ginger (grated)

• 1 tablespoon fresh turmeric (grated)

• Juice of 3-4 lemons

• 2-3 tablespoons honey or maple syrup (adjust to taste)

• Ice cubes

Instructions:

1. In a saucepan, bring water to a boil. Add grated ginger and turmeric. Simmer for 5-7 minutes. Let it cool.

2. In a pitcher, combine the cooled ginger turmeric infusion, freshly squeezed lemon juice, and honey or maple syrup. Stir well.

3. Refrigerate the lemonade until cold.

4. Pour the ginger turmeric lemonade over ice cubes in glasses and enjoy this refreshing and immune-boosting drink.

Berry Beet Smoothie

Ingredients:

• 1 small cooked beet (peeled and chopped)

• 1/2 cup mixed berries (strawberries, raspberries, blueberries)

• 1/2 cup unsweetened coconut water

• 1/2 cup Greek yogurt (unsweetened)

• Optional: 1 tablespoon honey or maple syrup

Instructions:

1. In a blender, combine cooked beet, mixed berries, coconut water, Greek yogurt, and honey or maple syrup if desired.

2. Blend until the mixture achieves a smooth consistency.

3. Pour the berry beet smoothie into a glass and enjoy this vibrant and antioxidant-rich beverage.

Minty Matcha Latte

Ingredients:

• 1 teaspoon matcha powder

• 1 cup unsweetened almond milk

- 1 teaspoon honey or maple syrup (optional)

- Fresh mint leaves for garnish

Instructions:

1. In a small saucepan, heat almond milk until warm (not boiling).

2. In a cup, whisk matcha powder with a small amount of warm almond milk until smooth.

3. Pour the rest of the warm almond milk into the cup with the whisked matcha and stir well.

4. Add honey or maple syrup for sweetness if desired. Stir until dissolved. Garnish with fresh mint leaves.

5. Enjoy this soothing minty matcha latte as a comforting and energizing beverage.

Carrot Apple Ginger Juice

Ingredients:

- 4 medium carrots (peeled and chopped)

- 2 apples (cored and chopped)

- 1-inch piece of fresh ginger (peeled)

• Optional: Splash of lemon juice

Instructions:

1. Wash, peel, and chop the carrots and apples. Peel the ginger.

2. Run the carrots, apples, and ginger through a juicer to extract the juice.

3. Add a splash of lemon juice for a tangy twist if desired.

4. Pour the freshly made carrot apple ginger juice into glasses and enjoy this vitamin-packed drink.

Hibiscus Iced Tea with Berries

Ingredients:

• 4 cups water

• 4 hibiscus tea bags

• 1 cup mixed berries (strawberries, raspberries, blueberries)

• Fresh mint leaves

• Ice cubes

Instructions:

1. Bring water to a boil. Add hibiscus tea bags and let them steep for about 5-7 minutes. Remove the tea bags and let the tea cool to room temperature.

2. Wash the mixed berries and tear a few mint leaves.

3. In a pitcher, place the mixed berries and torn mint leaves.

4. Pour the cooled hibiscus tea into the pitcher with the berries and mint. Refrigerate the infused tea until chilled.

5. Fill glasses with ice cubes and pour the hibiscus berry tea over the ice.

6. Optionally, garnish with additional fresh berries or mint leaves before serving.

Pineapple Ginger Mint Infused Water

Ingredients:

• Fresh pineapple chunks

• 1-inch piece of fresh ginger (peeled and sliced)

• Fresh mint leaves

• Ice cubes

• Water

Instructions:

1. Cut fresh pineapple into chunks. Peel and slice the ginger.

2. In a pitcher, combine the pineapple chunks, sliced ginger, and a few fresh mint leaves. Fill the pitcher with ice cubes and water.

3. Let the pitcher sit in the refrigerator for a few hours to infuse flavors.

4. Pour the pineapple ginger mint infused water into glasses, ensuring each serving has pineapple chunks, ginger slices, and mint leaves.

Melon Cucumber Mint Cooler

Ingredients:

• 2 cups cubed honeydew melon

• 1 cup cubed cucumber (peeled)

• Juice of 1 lime

• Fresh mint leaves

• Ice cubes

• Water or coconut water (optional)

Instructions:

1. In a blender, combine honeydew melon, cucumber, lime juice, and a few mint leaves.

2. Blend until the mixture turns smooth.

3. Optionally, strain the blended mixture through a fine-mesh sieve to remove pulp.

4. Refrigerate the drink to chill it further. Fill glasses with ice cubes and pour the melon cucumber mint cooler.

Blueberry Basil Sparkling Water

Ingredients:

• Fresh blueberries

• Fresh basil leaves

• Sparkling water

• Ice cubes

Instructions:

1. Wash the fresh blueberries and basil leaves.

2. In glasses, muddle a few blueberries and basil leaves gently to release flavors.

3. Fill the glasses with ice cubes and top them off with sparkling water. Stir the drink gently to combine flavors.

4. Enjoy the refreshing and subtly flavored blueberry basil sparkling water.

Mango Turmeric Smoothie

Ingredients:

- 1 ripe mango (peeled and cubed)

- 1/2 cup plain Greek yogurt (unsweetened)

- 1/2 teaspoon ground turmeric

- 1/2 teaspoon ground cinnamon

- 1 tablespoon honey or maple syrup (optional)

- 1/2 cup unsweetened almond milk or coconut water

Instructions:

1. In a blender, combine the ripe mango cubes, Greek yogurt, ground turmeric, ground cinnamon, honey or maple syrup (if using), and almond milk or coconut water.

2. Blend until the mixture becomes smooth and creamy.

3. Pour the mango turmeric smoothie into a glass and enjoy this vitamin-rich beverage.

Raspberry Lemon Verbena Iced Tea

Ingredients:

- 4 cups water

- 4 black tea bags

- 1 cup fresh raspberries

- Handful of fresh lemon verbena leaves (or mint leaves)

- Ice cubes

Instructions:

1. Boil water and steep black tea bags in the hot water according to package instructions. Let the tea cool to room temperature.

2. In a pitcher, muddle fresh raspberries and lemon verbena leaves gently to release flavors.

3. Pour the cooled black tea into the pitcher with the muddled raspberries and lemon verbena.

4. Refrigerate the tea until chilled. Fill glasses with ice cubes and pour the raspberry lemon verbena iced tea.

Kiwi Spinach Smoothie

Ingredients:

• 2 ripe kiwis (peeled and chopped)

• Handful of fresh spinach leaves

• 1/2 banana

• 1/2 cup unsweetened almond milk

• 1 tablespoon honey or maple syrup (optional)

Instructions:

1. In a blender, combine the chopped kiwis, fresh spinach leaves, banana, almond milk, and honey or maple syrup if desired.

2. Blend until the mixture turns into a smooth and green-hued drink.

3. Pour the kiwi spinach smoothie into a glass and relish this nutrient-packed beverage.

Cherry Mint Infused Water

Ingredients:

• Fresh cherries (pitted and halved)

• Fresh mint leaves

• Ice cubes

• Water

Instructions:

1. Pit and halve fresh cherries. Wash fresh mint leaves.

2. In a pitcher, combine the halved cherries and fresh mint leaves. Fill the pitcher with ice cubes and water.

3. Let the pitcher sit in the refrigerator for a few hours to infuse flavors.

4. Pour the cherry mint infused water into glasses, ensuring each serving has cherries and mint leaves.

Lemon Basil Sparkling Lemonade

Ingredients:

• Juice of 4-5 lemons

• Handful of fresh basil leaves

• 1/4 cup honey or maple syrup

• Sparkling water

• Ice cubes

Instructions:

1. Extract juice from the lemons. Wash and tear fresh basil leaves.

2. In a pitcher, combine the lemon juice, torn basil leaves, and honey or maple syrup. Muddle gently to infuse flavors.

3. Fill the pitcher with sparkling water and ice cubes. Stir well.

4. Pour the lemon basil sparkling lemonade into glasses and enjoy this refreshing drink.

Blueberry Lavender Lemonade

Ingredients:

• 1 cup fresh blueberries

• 4 cups water

• Juice of 3-4 lemons

• 2-3 tablespoons honey or maple syrup

• 1 tablespoon dried lavender flowers (culinary grade)

Instructions:

1. In a blender, blend fresh blueberries until smooth. Set aside.

2. In a saucepan, bring water to a boil. Remove from heat and add dried lavender flowers. Let it steep for 10-15 minutes. Strain and let it cool.

3. In a pitcher, mix the blueberry puree, strained lavender infusion, freshly squeezed lemon juice, and honey or maple syrup. Stir well.

4. Refrigerate the mixture until chilled.

5. Pour the blueberry lavender lemonade into glasses over ice cubes.

Mango Mint Green Tea

Ingredients:

- 2 cups hot water

- 2 green tea bags

- 1 ripe mango (peeled and diced)

- Handful of fresh mint leaves

- Optional: Honey or agave syrup (to taste)

Instructions:

1. Steep green tea bags in hot water for 3-4 minutes. Remove the tea bags and let it cool.

2. In a blender, combine diced mango and fresh mint leaves. Blend until smooth.

3. Mix the cooled green tea with the mango-mint puree. Add sweetener if desired and stir well.

4. Refrigerate the mango mint green tea until cold.

5. Pour over ice and garnish with additional mint leaves if desired.

Pineapple Basil Agua Fresca

Ingredients:

• 2 cups fresh pineapple chunks

• 4 cups water

• Juice of 2 limes

• Handful of fresh basil leaves

• Optional: Agave syrup or honey (to taste)

Instructions:

1. In a blender, combine fresh pineapple chunks, water, lime juice, and basil leaves. Blend until smooth.

2. Optionally, strain the mixture through a fine-mesh sieve to remove pulp.

3. Add agave syrup or honey to sweeten the agua fresca, if desired. Stir until dissolved.

4. Refrigerate the pineapple basil agua fresca until cold.

5. Pour into glasses over ice cubes and garnish with basil leaves.

Apple Cinnamon Oatmeal Smoothie

Ingredients:

• 1 apple (cored and chopped)

• 1/2 cup rolled oats

• 1/2 teaspoon ground cinnamon

• 1 cup unsweetened almond milk

• 1 tablespoon almond butter

• Optional: Honey or maple syrup (to taste)

Instructions:

1. In a blender, combine chopped apple, rolled oats, ground cinnamon, almond milk, and almond butter.

2. Blend until the mixture is smooth and oats are well incorporated.

3. Add honey or maple syrup for sweetness, if desired. Blend again until combined.

4. Pour the apple cinnamon oatmeal smoothie into glasses and enjoy.

Pomegranate Ginger Fizz

Ingredients:

- 1 cup pomegranate juice

- 2 cups sparkling water

- 1-inch piece fresh ginger (grated)

- Juice of 1 lime

- Optional: Honey or agave syrup (to taste)

- Ice cubes

Instructions:

1. In a pitcher, mix pomegranate juice, sparkling water, grated ginger, lime juice, and sweetener if desired. Stir well.

2. Refrigerate the mixture until cold.

3. Pour the pomegranate ginger fizz into glasses filled with ice cubes.

Peach Basil Iced Tea

Ingredients:

• 4 cups water

• 4 black tea bags

• 2 ripe peaches (pitted and sliced)

• Handful of fresh basil leaves

• Ice cubes

Instructions:

1. Boil water and steep black tea bags in the hot water according to package instructions. Let the tea cool to room temperature.

2. In a pitcher, muddle sliced peaches and fresh basil leaves gently to release flavors.

3. Pour the cooled black tea into the pitcher with the muddled peaches and basil. Refrigerate the tea until chilled.

4. Fill glasses with ice cubes and pour the peach basil iced tea.

Strawberry Rosemary Infused Water

Ingredients:

• Fresh strawberries (sliced)

• Fresh rosemary sprigs

• Ice cubes

• Water

Instructions:

1. Slice fresh strawberries and wash fresh rosemary sprigs.

2. In a pitcher, combine sliced strawberries and rosemary sprigs. Fill the pitcher with ice cubes and water.

3. Allow the pitcher to sit in the refrigerator for a few hours to infuse flavors.

4. Pour the strawberry rosemary infused water into glasses, ensuring each serving has strawberries and rosemary.

Coconut Berry Smoothie

Ingredients:

• 1 cup mixed berries (strawberries, blueberries, raspberries)

• 1/2 cup unsweetened coconut milk

• 1/2 cup Greek yogurt (unsweetened)

• 1 tablespoon unsweetened shredded coconut

• Optional: Honey or agave syrup (to taste)

Instructions:

1. In a blender, combine mixed berries, coconut milk, Greek yogurt, and shredded coconut.

2. Blend until the mixture reaches a smooth consistency.

3. Add honey or agave syrup for sweetness, if desired. Blend again until combined.

4. Pour the coconut berry smoothie into glasses and enjoy this tropical delight.

Turmeric Pineapple Ginger Elixir

Ingredients:

• 1 cup fresh pineapple chunks

• 1-inch piece fresh ginger (peeled)

• 1/2 teaspoon ground turmeric

• 1 tablespoon honey or maple syrup

• Juice of 1 lime

• 2 cups water

• Ice cubes

Instructions:

1. In a blender, combine fresh pineapple chunks, peeled ginger, ground turmeric, honey or maple syrup, lime juice, and water.

2. Blend until the ingredients form a smooth elixir.

3. Pour the turmeric pineapple ginger elixir over ice cubes and savor the refreshing drink.

Matcha Coconut Latte

Ingredients:

• 1 teaspoon matcha powder

• 1 cup unsweetened coconut milk

• 1 teaspoon honey or agave syrup

• Optional: Dash of vanilla extract

Instructions:

1. In a small saucepan, whisk matcha powder with a small amount of coconut milk until smooth.

2. Add the remaining coconut milk to the saucepan. Heat over medium-low heat, stirring occasionally.

3. Stir in honey or agave syrup. Add a dash of vanilla extract if desired.

4. Heat the mixture until hot but not boiling.

5. Pour the matcha coconut latte into a mug and enjoy this comforting beverage.

CONCLUSION

In conclusion, the Mind Diet stands as a nutritional approach that intertwines the principles of the Mediterranean Diet and the DASH (Dietary Approaches to Stop Hypertension) Diet, emphasizing the consumption of brain-boosting foods. With a foundation rooted in scientific research, this dietary pattern champions the incorporation of nutrient-rich foods like leafy greens, berries, nuts, whole grains, fish, and healthy fats, while advocating for the reduction of processed foods, red meats, and sugary items.

By prioritizing these wholesome foods, the Mind Diet not only supports brain health but also contributes to overall well-being. Its emphasis on specific nutrients, antioxidants, and healthy fats offers a promising approach to potentially reducing the risk of cognitive decline and neurodegenerative diseases.

Through its focus on fostering a balanced and diverse diet, the Mind Diet encourages individuals to adopt a sustainable and enjoyable way of eating. Its versatility allows for creativity in meal preparation, empowering individuals to savor delicious and nutritious meals while nurturing their cognitive health.

As we continue to delve deeper into understanding the intricate connection between nutrition and brain function, the Mind Diet remains a valuable guide, promoting not just a healthy body, but also a nourished and resilient mind. Incorporating the Mind Diet's principles into everyday life can serve as a meaningful step towards enhancing cognitive vitality and fostering a lifelong commitment to holistic health.

www.ingramcontent.com/pod-product-compliance
Lightning Source LLC
Chambersburg PA
CBHW050805260726
48660CB00004B/1270